TREATING IBD

A Patient's Guide to the Medical and Surgical

Management of Inflammatory Bowel Disease

TREATING IBD

A Patient's Guide to the Medical and Surgical Management of Inflammatory Bowel Disease

Editors

LAWRENCE J. BRANDT, MD.
Professor of Medicine
Albert Einstein College of Medicine
Director, Division of Gastroenterology
Montefiore Medical Center
Bronx, New York

PENNY STEINER-GROSSMAN, M.P.H.
Formerly Director of Research
and Education Programs
Crohn's & Colitis Foundation
of America, Inc.
New York, New York

Crohn's & Colitis Foundation of America, Inc.
(formerly the National Foundation for Ileitis and Colitis, Inc.)

Medical Illustrations by Ronald S. Futral

RAVEN PRESS 🐚 NEW YORK

Raven Press, 1185 Avenue of the Americas, New York, New York 10036

Made in the United States of America

Library of Congress Cataloging-in-Publication Data

Treating IBD.

   Includes bibliographical references.
    1. Ulcerative colitis—Treatment—Popular works.
2. Enteritis, Regional—Treatment—Popular works.
I. Brandt, Lawrence J.   II. Steiner—Grossman, Penny.
III. Crohn's & Colitis Foundation of America, Inc. (U.S.)
IV. Title.
RC862.C63T74   1989   616.3'447   87-42963
ISBN 0-88167-532-6 (soft)

9 8 7 6

This book is dedicated to the many people with inflammatory bowel disease and their families in the hope that it will add to an understanding of their disease, thereby lessening fear and anxiety.

Foreword

This book will not replace your physician or dictate how your IBD should be treated. Rather, the information in this book will make you a better informed patient who can understand what your doctor is doing and why. As your understanding grows, you will be able to ask better questions and become more involved in your care. A healthy relationship between you and your doctor is a very important part of your treatment.

Treating IBD is the latest in a series of informational efforts supported by the Crohn's & Colitis Foundation of America (CCFA). The CCFA has produced numerous brochures for patients, parents, and teachers, and two previous books, *The Crohn's Disease and Ulcerative Colitis Fact Book and People . . . not Patients.* Why another book? Because we want to provide the most current information available on the medical and surgical treatment of IBD. Some of the advances presented here are: new drug therapies, such as 5-ASA, 6-MP, and metronidazole; improvements in nutritional care; and recent surgical alternatives to ileostomy in ulcerative colitis, strictureplasty, and endoscopic balloon dilation of strictures in Crohn's disease.

We feel quite optimistic about the future. The therapy of Crohn's disease and ulcerative colitis is improving, and the scientific community and the many patients who participated in clinical research trials, have achieved milestones they can be proud of. Many of these studies were aided by CCFA research funds and, with ongoing research, we are confident there will be further advances. It is crucial that patients become aware of these accomplishments and it is our intention to help achieve this goal with this new publication.

Theodore M. Bayless, M.D.
Former Chairman, National Scientific Advisory Committee
Crohn's & Colitis Foundation of America, Inc.

Acknowledgments

We are deeply grateful to the many physicians and other professionals who made significant contributions to this book. In addition, we want to thank Marla Singer Gellerman and Shirley Howard, for their patience and perseverance in preparing the manuscript, Ronald S. Futral for his excellent illustrations, and June G. Rosenberg for preparing the index.

The publication of this book would not have been possible without the generous assistance of Sandoz Pharmaceuticals. With their help, we will be able to reach the many thousands of people with IBD who will benefit from the information in this book.

Lastly, we want to thank those patients with IBD from whom we have learned and continue to learn.

Lawrence J. Brandt
Penny Steiner-Grossman

This book was prepared under the auspices of the Crohn's & Colitis Foundation of America, Inc.

Contents

Part 3
When Surgery Becomes Necessary

Part 4
Operations for Ulcerative Colitis

Part 5
Operations for Crohn's Disease

Part 6
Special Surgical Situations

Contributors

Peter A. Banks, M.D.
Professor of Medicine
Tufts University School of Medicine
Chief, Division of Gastroenterology
St. Elizabeth's Hospital
736 Cambridge Street
Boston, Massachusetts 02135

Peter Barland, M.D.
Professor of Medicine
Albert Einstein College of Medicine
Acting Director, Division of
    Rheumatology
Montefiore Medical Center
111 East 210 Street
Bronx, New York 10467

Theodore M. Bayless, M.D.
Professor of Medicine
Johns Hopkins University School of
    Medicine
600 North Wolfe Street-Blalock 4
Baltimore, Maryland 21205

Jerrold M. Becker, M.D.
Professor of Clinical Surgery
State University of New York (Stony
    Brook)
Senior Attending Pediatric Surgeon
Schneider Children's Hospital, Long
    Island Jewish Medical Center
c/o 1300 Union Turnpike
New Hyde Park, New York 11040

Leslie H. Bernstein, M.D.
Professor of Medicine
Director, Unified Division of
    Gastroenterology

Montefiore Medical Center–Albert
    Einstein College of Medicine
111 East 210 Street
Bronx, New York 10467

Scott J. Boley, M.D.
Professor of Surgery and Pediatrics
Albert Einstein College of Medicine
Chief, Pediatric Surgical Services
Montefiore Medical Center
111 East 210 Street
Bronx, New York 10467

Lawrence J. Brandt, M.D.
Professor of Medicine
Albert Einstein College of Medicine
Director, Division of
    Gastroenterology
Montefiore Medical Center
111 East 210 Street
Bronx, New York 10467

Zane Cohen, M.D.
Associate Professor, Department of
    Surgery
University of Toronto
Surgeon, Division of General Surgery
Toronto General Hospital
101 College Street
Eaton Building 9-242
Toronto, Ontario, Canada M5G 1L7

Kiron M. Das, M.D., Ph.D.
Chief, Division of Gastroenterology
    and Hepatology
University of Medicine and Dentistry
    of New Jersey
Robert Wood Johnson Medical School
1 Robert Wood Johnson Place
New Brunswick, New Jersey 08903

Fredric Daum, M.D.
Professor of Clinical Pediatrics
Cornell University Medical College
Chief, Division of Pediatric
  Gastroenterology
North Shore University Hospital
300 Community Drive
Manhasset, New York 11030

George Dickstein, M.D.
Albert Einstein College of Medicine–
  Montefiore Medical Center
111 East 210 Street
Bronx, New York 10467

Douglas, A. Drossman, M.D.
Associate Professor of Medicine and
  Psychiatry
University of North Carolina
324 Clinical Sciences Building–
  229H
Chapel Hill, North Carolina 27514

Victor Fazio, M.D.
Chairman, Department of Colorectal
  Surgery
Cleveland Clinic Foundation
9500 Euclid Avenue
Cleveland, Ohio 44106

Gerald Friedman, M.D., Ph.D.
Associate Clinical Professor of
  Medicine
Mount Sinai School of Medicine
1 Gustave L. Levy Place
New York, New York 10029

Irwin M. Gelernt, M.D.
Clinical Professor of Surgery
Mount Sinai School of Medicine
1 Gustave L. Levy Place
New York, New York 10029

Donald J. Glotzer, M.D.
Associate Professor of Surgery
Harvard Medical School
Surgeon, Beth Israel Hospital
330 Brookline Avenue
Boston, Massachusetts 02215

Adrian J. Greenstein, M.D.
Professor of Surgery
Mount Sinai School of Medicine
1 Gustave L. Levy Place
New York, New York 10029

TennieBee M. Hall
Past President
United Ostomy Association, Inc.
c/o 5284 Dawes Street
San Diego, California 92109

Stephen B. Hanauer, M.D.
Associate Professor of Medicine
University of Chicago Medical Center
5841 South Maryland Avenue
Chicago, Illinois 60637

Henry D. Janowitz, M.D.
Clinical Professor of Medicine,
  Emeritus
Mount Sinai School of Medicine
1 Gustave L. Levy Place
New York, New York 10029

Marvin Kaplan, M.D.
Attending Psychiatrist
Lenox Hill Hospital
100 East 77 Street
New York, New York 10021

Keith A. Kelly, M.D.
Professor and Chairman, Department
  of Surgery
Mayo Medical School
200 First Street S.W.
Rochester, Minnesota 55901

Joseph B. Kirsner, M.D., Ph.D.
The Louis Block Distinguished
  Service Professor of Medicine
University of Chicago Medical Center
5841 South Maryland Avenue
Box 319
Chicago, Illinois 60637

Linda Klein, R.N., B.S.N., C.E.T.N.
Senior Clinical Research Associate
Marion Laboratories, Inc.
9300 Ward Parkway–East 3
Kansas City, Missouri 64114

Burton I. Korelitz, M.D.
Clinical Professor of Medicine
New York Medical College
Chief, Section of Gastroenterology
Lenox Hill Hospital
100 East 77 Street
New York, New York 10021

Ross S. Levy, M.D.
Assistant Professor of Medicine
(Dermatology)
Albert Einstein College of Medicine–
Montefiore Medical Center
111 East 210 Street
Bronx, New York 10467

Richard P. MacDermott, M.D.
Associate Professor of Medicine
Washington University School of
Medicine
660 South Euclid Avenue
Box 8124
St. Louis, Missouri 63110

Lester W. Martin, M.D.
Professor of Surgery and Pediatrics
Children's Hospital Medical Center
240 Bethesda Avenue
Cincinnati, Ohio 45229

Kevin Morrissey, M.D.
Clinical Associate Professor of
Surgery
Cornell Medical College—New York
Hospital
c/o 50 East 69 Street
New York, New York 10021

Peter A. Plumeri, D.O., LL.M.
Clinical Assistant Instructor in
Medicine
New Jersey School of Osteopathic
Medicine
c/o RD #1 Egg Harbor Road
Sewell, New Jersey 08080

Daniel H. Present, M.D.
Associate Clinical Professor of
Medicine
Mount Sinai School of Medicine
1 Gustave L. Levy Place
New York, New York 10029

Arvey I. Rogers, M.D.
Professor of Medicine
University of Miami School of
Medicine
Chief, Gastroenterology Section
Veterans Administration Hospital
c/o 8501 S.W. 87 Court
Miami, Florida 33173

William B. Ruderman, M.D.
Director of Gastroenterology
Cleveland Clinic Florida
3000 West Cypress Creek Road
Fort Lauderdale, Florida 33309

David B. Sachar, M.D.
Professor of Medicine
Mount Sinai School of Medicine
Director, Division of
Gastroenterology
Mount Sinai Medical Center
1 Gustave L. Levy Place
New York, New York 10029

Michael D. Sitrin, M.D.
Associate Professor of Medicine and
Committee on Human Nutrition and
Nutritional Biology
University of Chicago Medical Center
950 East 59 Street
Box 400
Chicago, Illinois 60637

Norman Sohn, M.D.
Clinical Assistant Professor of
Surgery
New York University School of
Medicine
c/o 475 East 72 Street
New York, New York 10021

Penny Steiner-Grossman, M.P.H.
Formerly Director of Research and
Education Programs
Crohn's & Colitis Foundation of
America, Inc.
444 Park Avenue South
New York, New York 10016
and
Freelance Health Writer
9 Prospect Park West (Apt. 9B)
Brooklyn, NY 11215

William F. Stenson, M.D.
Associate Professor of Medicine
Washington University School of
Medicine
Chief, Division of Gastroenterology
Jewish Hospital of St. Louis
660 South Euclid Avenue
Box 8124
St. Louis, Missouri 63110

Alan Uliss, M.D.
Assistant Professor Opthalmology
Albert Einstein College of Medicine–
Montefiore Medical Center
111 East 210 Street
Bronx, New York 10467

Malcolm C. Veidenheimer, M.D.
Staff, Department of Colon-Rectal
Surgery
Lahey Clinic Medical Center
41 Burlington Mall Road
Burlington, Massachusetts 01803

Edwina A. Zagami, B.S.N., M.Ed.
University of North Carolina
324 Clinical Sciences Building–
229H
Chapel Hill, North Carolina 27514

TREATING IBD

A Patient's Guide to the Medical and Surgical

Management of Inflammatory Bowel Disease

PART 1

Medical Management

1 / What Is Known about the Cause of IBD

The search for the cause of inflammatory bowel disease (IBD) has preoccupied IBD researchers for at least the past 50 years. Early investigators spent much time looking for and rejecting viruses and numerous types of bacteria as the probable initiators of the disease process. However, the recent discovery of a new bacterial species of the Mycobacterium family in the intestines of some patients with Crohn's disease is a promising new avenue of research in this area. The relative success of some antibacterial drugs—especially sulfasalazine and metronidazole—reinforces the belief that bacteria are somehow involved in the disease.

It is useful to remember that the intestine's thin inner lining allows certain intestinal contents to pass deep into the bowel wall. This suggests that irritating substances, for example the chemicals present in the outer coat or cell wall of many different types of bacteria, could leak through and set up the chronic inflammation that leads to IBD and to the immunologic changes that IBD patients manifest.

Whatever the "initiating event"—a bacterium, bacterial products, or a chemical or environmental agent—the initial acute inflammation becomes chronic and self-perpetuating in the genetically susceptible individual, and sets in motion a chain of destructive immunologic reactions (Fig. 1). These reactions, and the powerful substances and cells that regulate them, are the focus of intense scrutiny by most IBD researchers at work today. By understanding the particular inflammatory response seen in IBD, these researchers hope to work backward to discover the agent or event setting off this response.

WHAT HAPPENS DURING INFLAMMATION

The inflammatory response is the way in which our immune system rallies to attack infecting or damaging agents. The basic pattern is the same whether the offending agent is the streptococcus bacillus attacking the throat or the pollen that produces an asthmatic attack. The affected area becomes warm, reddened, painful, and swollen, and surrounding blood vessels become congested. Various cells, such as lymphocytes, leukocytes, mast cells, and macrophages, migrate to the inflamed area. While attacking the "invaders," these inflammatory cells release

3

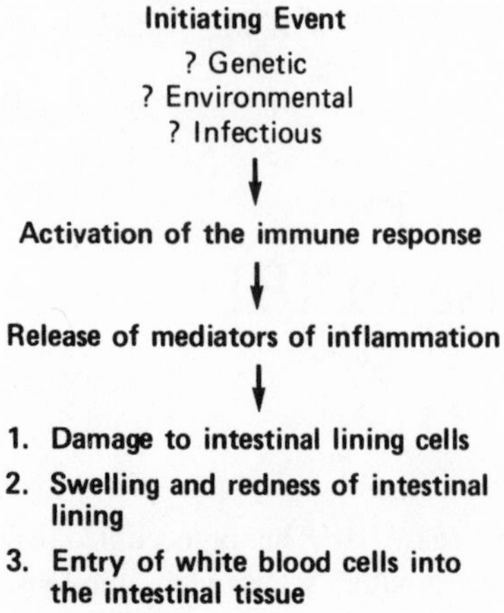

Initiating Event
? Genetic
? Environmental
? Infectious

↓

Activation of the immune response

↓

Release of mediators of inflammation

↓

1. **Damage to intestinal lining cells**
2. **Swelling and redness of intestinal lining**
3. **Entry of white blood cells into the intestinal tissue**

FIG. 1. A model for the inflammatory response in IBD.

powerful chemicals (inflammatory mediators), which also act as chemical "messengers" circulating in the blood to attract more inflammatory cells to the site.

Inflammation in the intestine has several hallmarks. In addition to the swelling, redness, and pain, there is damage to the intestinal lining (mucosa), creating a break in the protective mucosal barrier. Ulcerations form, and supporting cells and tissues may be exposed to intestinal bacteria and their harmful products as well as to enzymes released by the inflammatory cells. Blood and tissue fluid may leak from the intestinal wall, showing up as diarrhea or blood in the stool. The response by the body's inflammatory cells may cause even more damage than would have been caused by the original agent. In this case the immune response is "out of control," or self-perpetuating.

THE IMMUNE RESPONSE IN IBD

Although some scientists feel that the immune response observed in IBD is initiated by an unknown agent and perpetuated by leakage of bacterial products through the wounded bowel wall, others suggest that the inflammatory cells are reacting to the IBD patient's own tissues as if they were foreign, a process we know as autoimmunity. At the very least, we do know that certain specific immunologic disturbances have been found in persons with IBD. Correspondingly, the medications that are used to treat IBD are known to correct or inhibit many of these immunologic disturbances. For example, one of the actions of corticosteroids is blocking the synthesis of inflammatory mediators, such as prostaglandins and leukotrienes, which aggravate and perpetuate inflammations in IBD. The drug 5-aminosalicylic acid (5-ASA), the active component in sulfasalazine, also inhibits the production of inflammatory mediators and slows the production of harmful antibodies in the IBD patient. In addition, 5-ASA prevents the production of oxygen radicals—toxic compounds known to cause intestinal inflammation—thus interrupting the immunologic chain of events at several levels.

Thus it is clear that medications that interfere with the immune response and suppress inflammation are useful in treating ulcerative colitis and Crohn's disease. What remains is for IBD researchers to uncover the events leading to the initiation of the inflammatory response so that medications may one day cure IBD or prevent it altogether.

2//
What to Expect
from Medical Treatment

Until a cause is established, there can be no curative medical treatment either for ulcerative colitis or for Crohn's disease. None of the available medications exerts a "specific" pharmacologic or biologic effect, so current medical therapy for IBD attempts to control symptoms and eliminate the inflammatory reaction in the bowel. However, many patients respond to a program that includes a well-balanced, nutritious diet and the use of nonspecific medications. A variety of medications is available to ease abdominal pain or diarrhea, and to treat inflammation in the bowel. The judicious use of steroids, immunosuppressive drugs, and antimicrobial drugs may also be indicated at various times during the course of disease.

In general, the principles of treatment are similar for ulcerative colitis and for Crohn's disease, although there are some important differences. For example, ulcerative colitis is cured by removal of the colon and rectum, whereas Crohn's disease frequently recurs after surgery. Medical therapy is usually required for longer periods in Crohn's disease than in ulcerative colitis, in part because of the nature of the disease and in part because of the tendency for Crohn's disease to recur after operation. Crohn's disease is associated more commonly with nutritional deficiencies than ulcerative colitis because the small bowel is often involved and one or more intestinal resections may be required, thus interfering with absorption of nutrients. Complete nutritional evaluation and monitoring, therefore, while important in the management of IBD in general, is crucial for patients with Crohn's disease. Most physicians emphasize a program of treatment rather than just relying on one or two drugs.

GOALS OF IBD TREATMENT

The immediate goals of IBD therapy are the correction of nutritional deficiencies and the control of inflammation, with relief of abdominal pain, diarrhea, and rectal bleeding. However, not all bowel symptoms in a patient with IBD necessarily represent an exacerbation of either ulcerative colitis or Crohn's disease. Patients with IBD, just like everyone else, can develop diarrhea and cramps from viral or bacterial infections. Repeated examinations of the stools for bacterial pathogens and toxins are therefore necessary before embarking on complicated

IBD treatment plans. Long-range objectives of medical treatment are sustained control of bowel symptoms, the prevention and prompt treatment of complications, and the reestablishment of a reasonably healthy and satisfying life. Each person with IBD represents an individual challenge to the physician, involving both the art and the science of medicine. The most successful medical care usually is provided by the physician who is especially interested in the inflammatory bowel diseases, who understands their nature and also the "workings" of the gastrointestinal tract, and who is committed both to the careful supervision of the day-to-day details of treatment and to the humanistic aspects of medical care. You, the responsible patient who has faith and trust in the physician and who benefits from the treatment program, are, of course, the other equally important member of the team.

Removing Aggravating Influences

Together, you and your physician should try to identify factors that can aggravate or worsen IBD and, if possible, eliminate them. These include antibiotics, which may cause diarrhea or an "antibiotic associated colitis," stressful emotional situations, undernutrition, physical fatigue, the inexpert self-use of medication, and inadequate physician supervision. In addition, oral contraceptives occasionally cause a form of colitis resembling ulcerative colitis or Crohn's disease of the colon in young women. Intestinal infections including "food poisoning" and the "nonspecific" diarrhea associated with trips to countries lacking adequate sanitation can also precipitate or aggravate IBD.

How Does Medical Treatment Help?

Probably the most important benefit of effective medical management is to quiet the inflammatory process, and thereby strengthen host defenses and facilitate the regeneration of normal bowel tissue. Normalization of diseased tissues in IBD, if it occurs, does not happen until after prolonged control of the disease, which may take years; occasionally, substantial improvement occurs sooner. Control of symptoms rather than cure of the disease is the expectation of current medical treatment. However, sustained control of disease activity often allows significant slowing of the inflammatory process, promotes healing of the bowel, and leads to a better quality of life.

People with IBD understandably get discouraged when faced occasionally with the possibility of repeated hospitalization, long-term disability, economic deprivation, social isolation, and an uncertain future. However, despite the limitations of current treatment, most people respond favorably to careful, well-directed, long-term medical management. Furthermore, current pharmaceutical research is generating many new types of medications that will increase the specificity and effectiveness of IBD therapy in the near future (*See Chapter 9*).

Consenting to Drug Treatment

Once the diagnosis of IBD is established, your physician should take the time and effort to explain the therapeutic options to you. Too often, drug therapy is instituted with little or no discussion. Before starting drug treatment with corticosteroids, sulfasalazine, immunosuppressives, or other medications, it is critical for your physician to obtain your informed consent for therapy. Medications used in treating IBD require particular attention. Not only are these medications known to have frequent and occasionally serious side-effects, but they are generally used for long periods of time, thus increasing the chances of adverse reactions.

Your physician should explain why a certain medication is being prescribed as well as detail its benefits and mode of action, its risks and potential complications, and the alternatives to its use. You have a right to participate in decisions about your treatment and no treatment should be instituted without your informed consent (*See Chapter 21*).

3 // Nonspecific Medications and What They Accomplish

Abdominal pain and diarrhea are common symptoms in IBD which also may be present in many other gastrointestinal disorders. Such general symptoms can be treated in a nonspecific way without necessarily treating their primary cause. Thus, for example, diarrhea may respond to Kaopectate® or Lomotil®, regardless of whether it is caused by IBD, food poisoning, or viral gastroenteritis. Specific therapy can be withheld until deemed necessary.

ANTIDIARRHEAL AGENTS AND PAIN MEDICATIONS

These medications may be used as short-term therapy or to supplement the use of more specific drugs such as antiinflammatory agents. They must be monitored carefully, particularly if they contain narcotics, since their chronic use may predispose to toxic megacolon or lead to drug dependence.

The most effective of the antidiarrheal agents is deodorized tincture of opium (DTO), although it is not widely used anymore. The usual dose is 10 drops after every other stool, to a maximum of 30 drops daily. Paregoric in doses of 5 ml has an equivalent effect, and diphenoxylate (Lomotil®) or loperamide (Imodium®) is also quite effective. Codeine sulfate, in doses of 30 to 60 mg given every 4 to 6 hr, is favored by some physicians and might be preferable when abdominal pain is more of a problem than diarrhea.

Demerol® and Percocet® are also highly effective pain relievers. Aspirin products may be taken to alleviate pain when disease is inactive, but should be avoided during periods of active disease, since they inhibit platelet function and may increase the degree of bleeding from the bowel. It is important to remember that medications to relieve pain and diarrhea do just that; they do *not* treat the underlying inflammation which causes these symptoms. Subsequent chapters contain a complete discussion of specific therapeutic agents for IBD.

SEDATIVES AND TRANQUILIZERS

Phenobarbital, chlordiazepoxide (Librium®), diazepam (Valium®), alprazolam (Xanax®), or equivalent drugs are helpful in counteracting the insomnia and psy-

9

chic stimulation that may follow the introduction of high-dose steroids. If your physician prescribes these agents, he/she should monitor their use carefully, since they may cause lethargy or accentuate a preexisting depression.

DRUG DEPENDENCE

Drug dependence is the medical term for addiction. Dependence occurs most commonly with oral narcotics such a Percocet®, Percodan®, Demerol®, or Dilaudid® when these medications are prescribed for abdominal pain. Although these agents are quite effective at first, they become less effective after 2 to 4 weeks of regular use because the body develops a tolerance to them. For continued control of pain, the dose would then need to be increased; if this is done, a cycle is set up in which higher and higher doses become necessary. At some point, physical addiction develops and there are withdrawal symptoms if the narcotic is stopped. This cycle is much less common with narcotics such as codeine or Lomotil®, which are used to control diarrhea, since the potency and doses are lower than those used to control pain.

The best way to prevent drug dependence is not to use narcotics for long-term pain control. Every effort should be made to find a specific medical or surgical solution for the problem causing the pain. If this approach is not successful, there are physicians specializing in pain management who use nonaddictive drugs, hypnosis, biofeedback, and other techniques to help patients cope with pain. If narcotics must be prescribed for pain, they should be prescribed by only one physician who can closely monitor their use.

Special problems arise when a person with a potential drug or alcohol problem develops IBD. Since 6% of the population has a drug problem and another 6 to 9% has an alcohol problem, the physician caring for the IBD patient must know about these personal details.

ANTICHOLINERGIC AND ANTISPASMODIC DRUGS
(BENTYL®, PROBANTHINE®, DONNATOL®)

In general, this group of drugs should be avoided in the long-term management of IBD. Although anticholinergic drugs are occasionally useful in relieving abdominal cramps, they may cause atony (lack of muscle tone) of the bowel and contribute to small bowel obstruction or toxic megacolon when taken excessively.

ANTIBIOTICS

Of all the antibiotics, only metronidazole (Flagyl®) appears to have a specific action in IBD, that of closing perineal fistulas and improving the overall symptoms of Crohn's disease. Other antibiotics may be used on occasion to treat the secondary infections caused by perforations, abscesses, and fistulas in Crohn's disease. Occasionally, broad spectrum antibiotics such as ampicillin, cephalosporin (Keflex®), or tetracycline seem to improve the course of Crohn's disease after having been introduced for treatment of an infection or an abdominal mass. In these cases, extended use of antibiotics may be justified, although there are no controlled studies of these agents in IBD. Antibiotics are administered intravenously when disease is severe enough to require hospitalization, or when there is a complication such as toxic megacolon.

CHOLESTYRAMINE (QUESTRAN®)

Bile acids are normally secreted by the liver and then pass into the small intestine to aid in the absorption of fat. Most bile acids are then reabsorbed in the ileum and returned to the liver. After loss of the terminal portion of the ileum because of disease or surgical resection, the surface area available for reabsorption of the bile salts is reduced. Under these circumstances, the bile salts pass into the colon where they irritate the bowel and cause watery diarrhea. Cholestyramine acts by combining with the bile salts while they are still in the small intestine, forming an insoluble compound that does not irritate the colon and is excreted in the feces.

Cholestyramine can be dramatically effective in lessening the diarrhea that normally follows intestinal resection, and in treating the diarrhea in patients with extensive Crohn's disease who have not had surgery. It is available in powder form, either in individual packets or in bulk. The powder must be mixed with water or juice and should not be taken in dry form. It is usually administered 3 or 4 times daily before meals. Recently, cholestyramine became available in a flavored resin bar, under the name Cholebar®. Cholestyramine may interact with other drugs such as anticoagulants.

DIURETICS

Diuretics (Diuril®, Hydrodiuril®, Lasix®, Dyazide®) are often prescribed for individuals with IBD who have accummulated excess salt and water as a result of taking steroids. Diuretics should be used sparingly and only under your physician's direction. They can cause dehydration and excessive loss of essential electrolytes, such as potassium, leading to muscle weakness and even paralysis.

ANTACIDS AND H-2 BLOCKERS

Antacids are prescribed frequently for specific and nonspecific upper gastrointestinal symptoms such as pain, dyspepsia, or reflux (backflow of stomach acid) in patients with IBD. Since many antacids contain a magnesium product similar to that contained in the laxative Milk of Magnesia®, antacids can cause or worsen diarrhea. If an antacid is needed, a nonmagnesium-containing product such as Amphogel® or Basogel® may be preferred over Maalox®, Mylanta®, or other products containing magnesium.

H-2 blockers such as Zantac®, Tagamet®, and Pepcid® reduce the production of acid by the stomach and are commonly used in the treatment of peptic ulcer disease. They are also used to alleviate the symptoms of Crohn's disease of the stomach and duodenum, since these symptoms are often difficult to distinguish from ulcer disease. H-2 blockers are frequently prescribed along with steroids because some investigators feel that the incidence of ulcer formation is higher in those taking steroids than in other individuals. Although this cause and effect issue is controversial, physicians may prescribe antacids and/or H-2 blockers when steroids are given, simply to minimize the risk that ulcers may develop.

NONSTEROIDAL ANTIINFLAMMATORY DRUGS

Doctors have known for years that certain types of medications, called nonsteroidal antiinflammatory drugs (NSAIDs), used to treat arthritis may cause or aggravate stomach and duodenal ulcers and interfere with clotting.

Drugs in this category include indomethacin (Indocin®), naproxen (Naprosyn®), ibuprofen (Motrin®), and over-the-counter drugs such as aspirin and Advil® (ibuprofen in reduced strength). IBD patients who take these medications to relieve the joint pains associated with their disease should be aware that they may increase bleeding and also cause small intestinal inflammation (*See Chapter 10*). Considering the widespread use of these drugs, especially the over-the-counter preparations, it would seem reasonable that IBD patients use them with extreme caution, and under the careful scrutiny of the gastroenterologists, in relieving the arthritis symptoms associated with IBD.

4 / Sulfasalazine

When sulfa drugs were discovered during the 1930s, physicians began using them to treat many diseases felt to have an infectious cause. One such disease was rheumatoid arthritis, and in the 1940s Dr. Nana Svartz of Sweden began treating her rheumatoid patients with an antibacterial agent (sulfapyridine) and an antiinflammatory drug (salicylic acid). Ultimately, this led to the development of sulfasalazine (Azulfidine®), a single drug made up of sulfapyridine linked to 5-aminosalicylic acid (5-ASA) by a chemical bond (Fig. 1). In her clinical trials, Dr. Svartz observed that some patients with arthritis and ulcerative colitis showed surprising improvement in their colitis symptoms while taking sulfasalazine. Since this observation, sulfasalazine has become the standard therapy for mild to moderate IBD.

HOW SULFASALAZINE IS METABOLIZED IN THE BODY

After an oral dose of sulfasalazine, about 25% of the drug is absorbed from the small intestine. The remainder passes into the colon, where bacteria split the chemical bond and release the components, 5-ASA and sulfapyridine. The sulfapyridine molecule acts only as a "carrier" to deliver the active portion of sulfasalazine, 5-ASA, to the lower intestine. Without sulfapyridine, 5-ASA in its unprotected form would be absorbed rapidly in the stomach and upper small bowel before it could reach the colon.

Most of the sulfapyridine is absorbed and transported to the liver where it undergoes a variety of metabolic reactions before it is eventually excreted in the urine. As you will read later in this chapter, sulfapyridine is the portion of sulfasalazine that is responsible for most of the side effects caused by the parent drug. Individuals who excrete sulfapyridine slowly tend to accumulate it in the blood and are more likely to suffer side effects than are those who excrete it rapidly. The 5-ASA is not absorbed and therefore remains in contact with the inflamed colon before it is excreted in the stool.

SULFASALAZINE THERAPY IN IBD

Several randomized controlled trials have shown that sulfasalazine is effective in mild to moderate ulcerative colitis. About three-fourths of patients can be ex-

13

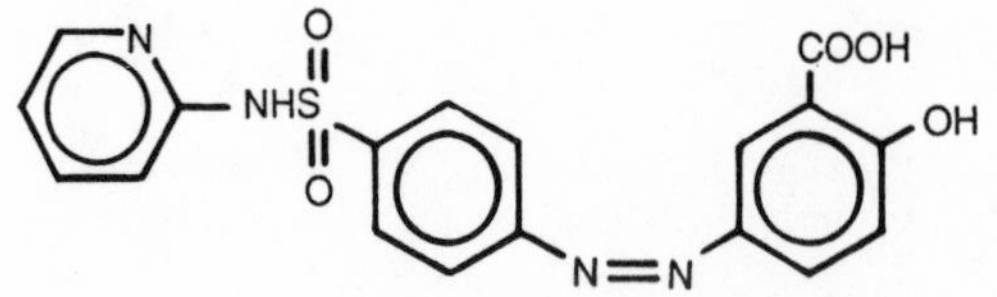

FIG. 1. Chemical structure of sulfasalazine.

pected to improve with sulfasalazine. However, during acute attacks, it appears that adjunctive steroid therapy is needed to achieve more rapid improvement. Several studies have shown that sulfasalazine is effective in delaying recurrences of ulcerative colitis, and a recent study demonstrated that close to 90% of patients with ulcerative colitis in remission who were given 2 gm/day of sulfasalazine remained symptom-free.

Early uncontrolled studies suggested that sulfasalazine was also useful in the treatment of Crohn's disease. In 1974, a double-blind controlled study involving a small number of subjects found the drug to be more effective than placebo in patients with active Crohn's disease who had had no prior surgery. Five years later, The National Cooperative Crohn's Disease Study (NCCDS) demonstrated that over a 4-month period, sulfasalazine was effective in patients with Crohn's colitis and ileocolitis; no benefit could be shown in patients with disease in the small bowel alone. In contrast to its use in ulcerative colitis, sulfasalazine has *not* been shown to be helpful in maintaining remission in Crohn's disease no matter where the disease is located.

Sulfasalazine is usually recommended as the initial treatment in patients with mild to moderate ulcerative colitis or with Crohn's disease involving the colon. The usual dose is 3 to 4 gm/day (6 to 8 tablets). At higher doses, side effects are more likely to occur. Therapy with sulfasalazine can be continued at a dose of 1.5 to 2 gm/day (3 to 4 tablets) in patients who have achieved remission.

It is still unclear why sulfasalazine has a beneficial effect in treating IBD. Although the drug may have some antibacterial effects, most researchers believe it is probably an antiinflammatory agent that blocks the production of certain harmful chemicals released in the intestine, called inflammatory mediators. Treatment with sulfasalazine also results in improved transport of sodium and water in the colon, and this may have an antidiarrheal effect as well. In addition, sulfasalazine may have immunosuppressive properties that remain to be investigated.

SIDE EFFECTS OF SULFASALAZINE

Although sulfasalazine is an essential drug for the treatment of IBD, about 20% of those who use it may experience a variety of side effects. Some of these side effects, such as rash, fever, and hepatitis, appear during the initial weeks of treatment, and are caused by an allergic or hypersensitivity reaction. These adverse reactions disappear when treatment is stopped. It is not uncommon in such situations, especially with skin rashes, to restart therapy with small doses of the drug and gradually to "desensitize" the patient (see below).

Most of the other side effects seem to be dose related, and include nausea, vomiting, dizziness, lack of appetite, headache, and joint pains. Sulfasalazine can also cause abnormalities in the sperm and a low sperm count, which leads to temporary infertility in men. This condition is reversible, and disappears when the drug is stopped. Sulfasalazine also can cross the placenta during pregnancy, raising concerns about its effects on the fetus, including possible jaundice in the newborn. In several large studies of women taking sulfasalazine during pregnancy, jaundice was not more common in babies whose mothers were taking sulfasalazine than it was in the control population. Most physicians no longer feel that sulfasalazine need be discontinued during pregnancy if it is necessary to control the symptoms of IBD. However, since sulfasalazine is excreted in breast milk, the drug is best not used if the mother is breast feeding. (A more complete discussion of the use of sulfasalazine and other drugs before and during pregnancy appears in Chapter 13). Because of the way it is metabolized by the body, sulfasalazine also may prevent the proper absorption of dietary folic acid (one of the B vitamins) from the small intestine. If folic acid deficiency occurs, your physician will advise you to take a folic acid supplement that will correct the problem.

Sulfasalazine may prevent the normal formation in the bone marrow of red blood cells, white blood cells, and platelets, resulting in severe deficiencies of these elements. Fortunately, these reactions are extremely rare and can be diagnosed quickly with a complete blood count (CBC) performed soon after the drug is started.

DESENSITIZATION

Many of the side effects of sulfasalazine can be minimized or prevented altogether through the use of gradually increasing doses of the medication, a process known as desensitization. After sulfasalazine is stopped for a week or two, side effects usually subside, and your physician may restart the drug, using very small doses ranging from 1 to 250 mg daily. Doses under 125 mg are difficult to prepare using available tablets, but are easy to measure out using the liquid form of the drug.

5 // Corticosteroids

Corticosteroids are widely used in the treatment of IBD because of their antiin-flammatory activity and their ability to suppress acute attacks of both Crohn's disease and ulcerative colitis. However, when a physician suggests their use, it often arouses much anxiety in both patients and family, since most people have heard of the drug's numerous side effects; parents, especially, may be concerned that the use of steroids will delay growth in their ill children. So it is crucial to put these important medications in perspective, and to weigh their risks against their potential benefits to the person with IBD.

STEROIDS AND ADRENOCORTICOTROPIC HORMONES (ACTH)

Corticosteroids are substances that resemble the hormones secreted daily from the outer rim (cortex) of the adrenal glands located at the top of the kidneys. These secretions have an effect on every cell in the body, and are necessary in minute amounts to maintain life. Indeed, if the normal adrenal glands fail to secrete steroid hormones, a potentially fatal condition called Addison's disease will result. The best known of the synthetic steroids is prednisone (Fig. 1). A similar drug is methylprednisolone (Medrol®). Both substances resemble the compound cortisol secreted by the adrenal gland, and in IBD are used to supplement the body's own steroids.

An alternative to steroid supplementation is the use of a substance called adrenocorticotropic hormone (ACTH), which stimulates the patient's adrenal gland to secrete its own steroids. ACTH is manufactured in the pituitary gland located at the base of the brain and travels through the blood stream to the adrenal gland, where it stimulates release of cortisol. In using ACTH to treat IBD, the physician attempts to mimic and amplify the way the body's hormone system normally works.

There are advantages and disadvantages to both forms of steroid treatment. The advantage of using prednisone is that it can be given by mouth and is easily absorbed in the intestine. ACTH cannot be taken orally but must be injected into the body either by intramuscular or intravenous injection. A major disadvantage of prednisone is that it suppresses normal adrenal gland function and thus *cannot* be

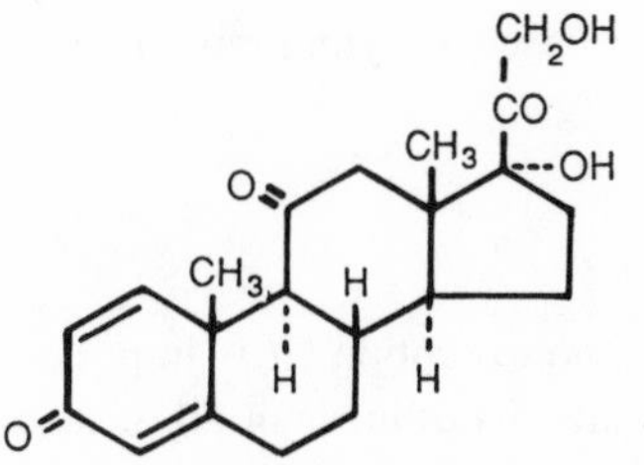

FIG. 1. Chemical structure of prednisone.

stopped abruptly. The adrenal glands need a period of days to weeks to recover from this suppression and return to normal patterns of daily secretion. The daily dose of prednisone is therefore gradually tapered over time rather than discontinued suddenly. On the other hand, ACTH stimulates the adrenals that do not "hibernate" under its effect, so this agent can be stopped abruptly if necessary.

Whether you are being treated with supplemental steroids or with ACTH, it is important to remember that the purpose of these drugs is to suppress inflammation in the intestine. Steroids are not given because your body does not make enough cortisone by itself. Also, these medicines are not believed to treat the cause of IBD, since that remains unknown. Rather, they act on the whole complicated chain of biochemical and tissue changes that produce inflammation in the body, and also interfere with any associated immunologic reactions. The simplest way to describe the actions of steroids and ACTH is to label them as "antiinflammatory drugs," and to distinguish them from the nonsteroidal antiinflammatory drugs (NSAIDs) used, for example, in treating chronic arthritis.

Effects of Steroids

The most important and desirable effect of steroids is suppression of intestinal inflammation and all its manifestations: pain, fever, loss of appetite, weakness, fatigue, abdominal tenderness, and bleeding from inflamed tissues. Steroids and ACTH also are used to suppress those disturbances that occur outside the intestine, referred to as the extraintestinal manifestations of IBD. These include inflammation of the eye (iritis and conjunctivitis), the skin (erythema nodosum and pyoderma gangrenosum), arthritis, and jaundice caused by inflammation and scarring in the bile ducts of the liver.

Although the antiinflammatory effects of steroids help you combat the specific symptoms of IBD, other effects are "nonspecific." For example, appetite is stimulated by the direct action of steroids on the brain. Similarly, taking steroids may improve the mood and impart a sense of well-being, the result of the action of these drugs on the emotional centers of the brain. Despite their ability to impart a sense of well-being, steroids may mask severe disease. Because of this and the many complications of steroids, their use should be monitored carefully by your physician. It is important to remember that steroids are used in *response* to symptoms of IBD and are not effective in preventing the onset of symptoms of either Crohn's disease or ulcerative colitis.

Side Effects

Every medication has side effects and steroids are no exception. It is important to remember that although some steroid side effects are disturbing, not all of them are dangerous, and most disappear gradually after the drug is discontinued.

Steroids do not provoke an allergic reaction; in fact, they are a recognized treatment for some allergic conditions, such as asthma. Steroids can disturb the day-night rhythm of the brain and lead to sleeplessness, especially if taken late in the day or just before bedtime. They also cause fluid retention and swelling of the face, hands, abdomen, and ankles. Since salt (sodium chloride) increases fluid retention, it is a good idea to avoid table salt and foods containing large amounts of sodium. The indiscriminate use of diuretics ("water pills") to get rid of this retained water should be avoided, whereas judicious use of these agents can be quite effective in making you more comfortable.

Steroids also cause some well known and unpleasant cosmetic effects that eventually disappear when the drug is stopped. The face may become rounded and "moon"-shaped, women may develop light downy hair on the face, and both sexes may develop facial acne that usually responds to standard treatment. Hair loss occurs occasionally but is more often caused by the underlying illness than by steroids. Treating the scalp is usually of no help, and hair growth will resume when the symptoms improve and the dose of steroids is reduced.

Since steroids also cause a rise in blood sugar, patients with diabetes may find that their diabetic control needs adjusting while they are taking these drugs. If you have a family history of diabetes, and your blood sugar rises while you are on steroid therapy, it is appropriate to be concerned; however, this alone should not cause you to discontinue steroids if they are necessary to control your symptoms.

The more serious side effects of steroids need more discussion. Mood swings, irritability, crying spells, distortions of personality, and even a "nervous breakdown" may be precipitated by high doses of steroids. If this happens, your physician will reduce the dose or discontinue the drug altogether, substituting other medications and offering psychological support. Some patients complain of heartburn while on steroids, but it is uncertain whether the drugs can cause a true "peptic" ulcer of the stomach or duodenum. They do cause irritation to the stomach lining, however, and may stir up a tendency to ulcers or activate an old ulcer. Some physicians prescribe antacids or one of the newer antiulcer medications to help prevent the development of ulcers (*See Chapter 3*). These medications may be helpful and they usually cause no harm.

Softening of the bones, especially of the spine (osteoporosis), is among the most serious side effects of steroid therapy, occurring only after prolonged use. Since people with IBD often avoid milk and dairy products, it is probably worthwhile to supplement the diet with calcium, especially if you are a woman with a tendency to develop osteoporosis.

Another severe bone problem occurring with prolonged use of high-dose steroids is osteonecrosis or aseptic necrosis. This serious condition typically affects the hips and wrists and causes severe pain. Although conventional x-rays may reveal advanced disease, computed tomography (CT) scans may enable earlier diagnosis. Unfortunately, there is no effective medical treatment for this condition and hip replacement may be necessary.

The question of whether steroids can slow the growth of children may be a difficult one to answer in an individual patient, since the disease itself is often the *primary* reason for delay in growth and sexual maturation. However, most physicians feel that the beneficial effects of steroids outweigh their harmful effects on growth and that steroids should be given a trial in children with IBD. One way to minimize possible adverse effects on growth is to administer steroids on alternate days, if possible. General experience confirms the rule that most children will have a "catch up" growth spurt no matter which form of treatment they undergo—medical or surgical—once the IBD is in prolonged remission.

After this catalog of the side effects of steroid therapy, you may wonder if they should be used at all. Steroids are extremely useful drugs and their side effects, although significant, should not lead us either to abandon them or to refuse to use them. If care is taken, their side effects can usually be well controlled or lessened and your symptoms improved immensely.

AVAILABLE FORMS OF STEROID DRUGS

Prednisone and methylprednisolone (Medrol®) are usually prescribed in tablet form. Hydrocortisone-containing suppositories, enemas (Cortenema®, Medrol-Enpak®), and foamy aerosols (Cortifoam®) are available for rectal use. Many patients who cannot retain steroid enemas prefer the foams, which are also convenient for traveling since the multidose package they come in is small and fits easily into a purse or pocket. If you are in the hospital and require steroids, they are usually given intravenously in the form of hydrocortisone (Solu-Medrol®). Regardless of the form in which steroids are given, they are absorbed into the body and are capable of causing side effects and of suppressing the normal steroid output of the adrenal glands. However, only about 20% of steroids administered through the rectum is absorbed and therefore the side effects mentioned earlier are seen less often with rectal than with oral preparations. A new form of steroid currently being developed, tixocortal pivalate, produces even fewer systemic effects and may represent an eventual solution to the problem of systemic toxicity of steroids.

When Are These Different Forms Used?

When bowel inflammation is just within the anus or the first few inches of the rectum, suppositories or foam preparations are often quite effective in relieving rectal symptoms such as pain, local bleeding, and urgency. If inflammation extends upward into the left side of the colon, either foam or the enema form of steroids is usually effective. Rectal preparations should be given slowly while you are lying on your back or left side. If you cannot hold the higher volume liquid enema, foam preparations are usually tolerated better and should be used initially. When administered this way, the enemas actually can reach much farther up the left side of the colon and may be retained for longer periods.

When disease is mild to moderate and involves the small intestine or the right side of the colon, which cannot be reached with enema preparations, steroids must be given orally. If symptoms are severe and you are hospitalized, you will probably receive hydrocortisone intravenously.

In the present-day treatment of IBD, the precise role of ACTH is unclear. It is a useful medication when the physician does not want to suppress the adrenal gland, and is of less value if the adrenal gland has been partially suppressed by previous steroid therapy. Some physicians suggest its use in sick patients who have either not responded to steroids or have not been on steroids in the recent past.

GETTING OFF STEROIDS

Since the severity of steroid side effects depends on the dose given and the duration of therapy, most physicians strive to reduce the dose and finally wean their patients from steroids. This *cannot* be done abruptly, but by slowly decreasing doses daily or weekly, the castastrophic effects of sudden withdrawal can be avoided. You should learn to recognize some of the milder symptoms of steroid reduction: yawning, "goose flesh," and muscular aches and pains. Because most patients feel so much better on steroids, they may be reluctant to come off them completely, especially if at the lower doses they still have some symptoms of bowel disease. If at all possible, it is better to accept the inevitability of some symptoms and be off the drugs than to insist on complete relief from every ache and pain and to remain on steroids indefinitely.

MAINTENANCE THERAPY

Maintenance therapy with any drug is essentially an attempt to prevent recurrences and to lessen their severity with the continued use of medication. However, steroids have not been shown to be effective in maintaining remission, either in Crohn's disease or ulcerative colitis. Sometimes, small doses of prednisone are necessary to promote well-being, but long-term use of prednisone should be avoided if possible.

6/ Metronidazole

Metronidazole (Flagyl®) is a potent antibiotic drug used to treat a variety of infections caused by anaerobic bacteria. This group of organisms is able to live only in places in which oxygen is virtually absent, such as the colon and rectum. Metronidazole is also effective against certain parasites, such as trichomonas which occur in the vagina, and the ameba, which can cause a type of colitis unrelated to IBD.

METRONIDAZOLE AS TREATMENT FOR CROHN'S DISEASE

In 1975, Dr. Bo Ursing at University Hospital in Lund, Sweden prescribed metronidazole to 5 patients with Crohn's disease. Dr. Ursing's rationale in using metronidazole was to reduce bacterial overgrowth in the small intestine and thereby improve absorption of nutrients. He also hoped to eliminate bacterial antigens that might be playing a role in causing disease. Four of his patients responded within 2 to 4 weeks and the fifth responded quite well within 4 months. Since Dr. Ursing first used the drug in 1975, thousands of patients have received metronidazole as treatment for Crohn's disease or, more specifically, for its perineal complications. Although recent investigators have not reported results quite so dramatic as those of Dr. Ursing, it is clear from controlled studies that metronidazole represents a treatment option for people with Crohn's colitis and especially for those with perineal involvement.

In all of the reports appearing after Dr. Ursing's pioneering work, it was noted that most patients with perineal manifestations of Crohn's disease seemed to benefit from metronidazole regardless of whether their intestinal symptoms improved (*See section on perineal disease in Chapter 10*). In one study of patients with perineal disease (e.g., fissures, fistulas, ulcers, and abscesses) resistant to conventional forms of therapy, about 80% improved while on the drug. Some patients were unable to continue the drug because of side effects and a few patients failed to respond. Metronidazole has also been shown to be an effective treatment for Crohn's disease of the colon, and in one controlled study was as useful as sulfasalazine.

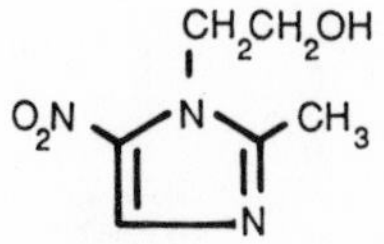

CH$_2$CH$_2$OH

O$_2$N　N　CH$_3$

N

FIG. 1. Chemical structure of metronidazole.

Metabolism and Safety

Metronidazole is absorbed very rapidly from the intestine and finds its way into all the body fluids, appearing within minutes on the mucous membranes of the mouth, intestinal tract, and genitourinary system (Fig. 1). Once in the body, it is broken down by the liver to several other compounds. Bacteria metabolize metronidazole differently, causing it to be more toxic to the bacteria than to you.

Several of the compounds resulting from the metabolism of metronidazole have been shown to produce genetic changes in bacterial test systems. However, mutations have *not* been demonstrated in humans tested with metronidazole or its breakdown products. In addition, no abnormalities in fetuses or infants have yet occurred when women have been given short courses of metronidazole during pregnancy. Nonetheless, the drug has yet to be proved harmless to the developing fetus and is best avoided during pregnancy. Metronidazole is excreted in the breast milk and therefore should not be taken by nursing mothers.

Despite numerous experiments showing that metronidazole and its metabolites cause a variety of tumors in laboratory animals, several large series have failed to show that metronidazole is capable of inducing tumors in patients treated with short courses of the drug. However, when metronidazole is given for Crohn's disease, it is usually prescribed for periods of several months or longer, and thus more experience is needed. The few cancers that have developed in patients on metronidazole therapy probably represent a coincidence and are not related to medical treatment.

Side Effects

Metronidazole has many side effects, some that are minor and one that is major. Among the minor side effects is a metallic taste in the mouth that may be associated with nausea and with a decrease in appetite (anorexia). Metronidazole may occasionally cause a sore throat or "furry" tongue, which is the result of changes in the bacterial population of the mouth. Dark urine is common but nothing to be concerned about. Headache, skin rashes, and hives are other minor side effects. All these minor adverse effects are short-lived and disappear quickly after the drug is discontinued.

When metronidazole is used for long periods of time, many patients will develop a numbness in the feet and lower legs. These unpleasant sensations, known as paresthesias, are annoying but rarely disabling. Some individuals note a feeling of coldness in the feet and hands, particularly in the winter months. Even when metronidazole is stopped, the numbness and paresthesias may persist for many months. Ultimately, these effects will disappear. Unfortunately, perineal disease tends to recur when metronidazole is stopped. The drug can be restarted when the paresthesias have improved or cleared and the initial good response can be expected. Some people have found the paresthesias of minor inconvenience when compared with the disability produced by the disease, and have chosen to live with the numb feelings and continue the drug. In any case, your physician will help you to decide whether or not to start or to continue metronidazole. It is important that you be observed closely by your doctor while taking this drug.

7 // Immunosuppressive Medications

The use of immunosuppressive agents such as 6-mercaptopurine (6-MP; Purine-thol®) and azathioprine (Imuran®) in the therapy of IBD is controversial. The two agents are chemically similar to one another, and actually, azathioprine is converted by the body into 6-MP (Fig. 1). Since the first reported use of immunosuppressive agents to treat ulcerative colitis in 1962, there have been numerous reports in the medical literature of their effectiveness. However, two major factors still cause reluctance in using them to treat patients with IBD. The first is the lack of numerous double-blind, controlled trials of immunosuppressives in IBD, and the second is fear of toxicity.

Double-blind, controlled trials allow researchers to look objectively at the effectiveness and safety of the drug being tested. (The subject of proper study design is discussed in Chapter 8.) Unfortunately, in Crohn's disease there have been only eight controlled trials using 6-MP or azathioprine, and only three controlled trials studying their use in ulcerative colitis. Many of these trials have used small numbers of patients treated for short periods of time, both of which are severe drawbacks in study design.

In uncontrolled studies in which these agents have been given directly to patients with Crohn's disease or ulcerative colitis, they have been shown to be effective in approximately 75% of cases.

IMMUNOSUPPRESSIVE AGENTS AND CROHN'S DISEASE

In patients with Crohn's disease, this degree of response has not been shown consistently in controlled studies. In fact, in one large study, the National Cooperative Crohn's Disease Study (NCCDS) in 1979, it was reported that azathioprine was *not* statistically more effective than placebo, in contrast to another controlled study that showed that 6-MP improved symptoms in 67% of patients with Crohn's disease. An explanation for this difference might be that azathioprine and 6-MP are not actually the same drugs; another possible explanation is that it takes these medications at least 3 to 6 months to take effect. In many controlled studies including the NCCDS, the drug was not used for this long a period, and these studies may have failed to demonstrate the drug's effectiveness for lack of time.

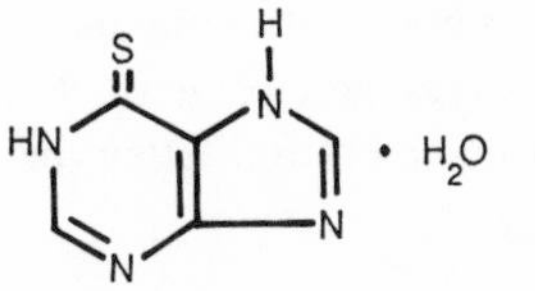

FIG. 1. Chemical structure of 6-mercaptopurine.

How then are you and your physician to decide whether immunosuppressives might be helpful? The evidence suggests strongly that 6-MP and azathioprine are effective in approximately two-thirds of patients. These drugs appear to work best when the colon is involved, but they also work when the small intestine is diseased. When given together with steroids, they often act in a "steroid-sparing" manner, allowing the physician to reduce or discontinue the dose of oral steroids once the immunosuppressives take effect. This steroid-sparing effect is most often relied on in the patient who has been on steroids for a long period of time or who has severe steroid side effects, such as diabetes, osteoporosis, or emotional problems. Immunosuppressives also heal or improve fistulas such as rectovaginal fistulas and fistulas from the intestine to other organs, such as the bladder or skin, in approximately 60% to 70% of patients.

In patients with severe Crohn's colitis or ileitis, or in those with recurrent disease or total colectomy and ileostomy, it is reasonable to try immunosuppressives in order to avoid surgery or to decrease the amount of bowel that might have to be removed. However, it is currently impossible to predict whether immunosuppressives can prevent a recurrence of Crohn's disease.

There are two controversial trials showing that immunosuppressives may act as "preventive agents" in Crohn's disease. These studies demonstrate that if patients improve on immunosuppressives and remain on these drugs, they will stay in remission more than 90% of the time. When drugs were stopped after 1 year, the relapse rate was approximately 80% in the next year. This study implied that if treatment is begun with immunosuppressives, you should probably take them for a minimum of 2 to 3 years.

IMMUNOSUPPRESSIVE AGENTS AND ULCERATIVE COLITIS

In ulcerative colitis, there have been only three controlled trials of immunosuppressives, involving only about 90 patients. One trial showed that immunosuppressives were effective, the second showed they were not, and the third reported that "clinical results with azathioprine can be judged to be encouraging but not definitely proved." Just as with Crohn's disease, uncontrolled reports in ulcerative colitis show that immunosuppressives are effective in about 75% of patients. Many physicians feel that since removing the colon is a cure for the disease, a potentially toxic drug should not be used. However, short-term use of immunosuppressives might be considered in a person with ulcerative colitis who is not acutely ill, and who is neither at high risk for developing cancer nor steroid intolerant. It also might be appropriate to use these agents to treat severe proctosigmoiditis, when total colectomy would be considered too radical a treatment for active disease limited to the lower colon.

Toxicity of Immunosuppressive Agents

The second factor discouraging the use of immunosuppressives has been the fear of toxicity, both short- and long-term. Both 6-MP and azathioprine have been used for many years to prevent the rejection of transplanted organs, and a great deal of information has been accumulated about toxicity of these agents. However, because of differences in doses and other factors, side effects that occur in transplant patients may not occur in patients with IBD. Therefore, we have only a few studies to rely on to help us determine the short- and long-term potential toxicity of immunosuppressives in IBD.

Allergy

There are several types of allergic reaction to immunosuppressive agents. Some individuals may develop a rash with or without fever and joint pains within a few weeks of starting treatment. This kind of allergic reaction is similar to what might be seen in someone who is allergic to penicillin. If this type of allergy develops after taking 6-MP, a similar reaction to azathioprine is likely, and neither drug should be used. When the medication is stopped, these allergic reactions will disappear completely.

Another type of reaction is pancreatitis, an inflammation of the pancreas. Pancreatitis causes pain in the abdomen and upper back pain, nausea, vomiting, and fever. These symptoms usually begin within 3 weeks of the start of immunosuppressive therapy and disappear promptly when the drug is stopped. In rare instances, immunosuppressives may cause allergic hepatitis, resulting in jaundice. As with pancreatitis, these symptoms are recognized quickly and disappear when the drug is stopped.

Infections

Since immunosuppressive medications reduce the number of white blood cells and other cells that fight infection in the body, physicians are concerned that their patients might develop infections while taking 6-MP or azathioprine. In a study of 400 patients taking 6-MP, the occurrence of severe infections was less than 2%. There were few unusual types of infections seen in this study, such as cytomegalovirus, but IBD patients occasionally develop such infections without ever taking immunosuppressives. The dosage of immunosuppressives used in IBD is quite a bit lower than that used in transplant patients, and probably results in less immunosuppression. How much immunosuppression is needed to achieve a good result is not known.

Development of Tumors

Early in the use of immunosuppressives for kidney transplant patients there was a high incidence of lymphomas, tumors of the blood-forming organs, and lymph nodes. In two large studies of IBD patients taking immunosuppressives, only 1 patient in more than 700 treated patients has developed a lymphoma. The exact incidence of lymphoma in IBD *without* immunosuppressive therapy is unknown, but recent studies at a number of medical centers have demonstrated that patients with Crohn's disease and possibly those with ulcerative colitis do have an increased incidence of leukemias and lymphomas. The fact that lymphomas and other tumors are not often seen in IBD patients taking immunosuppressives may be related to the lower doses being used. It remains to be seen if these patients will develop tumors if they continue to take low-dose immunosuppressives for long periods of time.

Sterility and Birth Defects

Another great concern of patients on these medications is that they may not have normal, healthy children. Although animal studies suggest that immunosuppressives can cause sterility and birth deformities, these defects are not seen when immunosuppressives are used in IBD patients or in those undergoing kidney transplant. As a precaution, however, physicians routinely advise that immunosuppressives be stopped before conception. However, a few patients with IBD unwittingly were taking the drug at the time of conception and many kidney transplant patients have taken the drug not only at conception but throughout pregnancy. No significant abnormalities have been reported in the children of these individuals.

CYCLOSPORINE (SANDIMMUNE®)

Studies are now underway with the newest immunosuppressive agent, cyclosporine. This agent has replaced azathioprine and 6-MP in treating most organ transplant patients. In fact, the use of cyclosporine to prevent organ rejection has greatly improved the success of liver and heart transplants. It is logical that if cyclosporine is a better immunosuppressive for transplant patients, then perhaps the drug might also be more effective in treating IBD. Preliminary data indicate that cyclosporine is effective and does work more rapidly than 6-MP or azathioprine to relieve the symptoms of intractable Crohn's disease. However, its effect may be shorter lasting than azathioprine and 6-MP, and it has serious side effects and possible long-term toxicities that may preclude its frequent use in IBD. It may take another 3 to 5 years to find out whether cyclosporine is worth the risk of its use in patients with IBD.

In summary, immunosuppressives appear to be effective in the treatment of IBD, but information on large numbers of patients treated for long periods of time is still lacking. Although only a small percent of patients with IBD should be considered for therapy with these drugs, those who are should fit within strict criteria. An open discussion with the physician about risks and the benefits of therapy with these agents should precede their use.

8 Testing New Drugs for IBD

You have already read that in the 1940s a Swedish physician, Dr. Nana Svartz, treated her rheumatoid arthritis patients with a combination of sulfapyridine and salicylate. Dr. Svartz observed that some of the patients with rheumatoid arthritis also suffered from ulcerative colitis and, occasionally, one or both conditions improved with therapy. These uncontrolled observations stimulated an American physician, Dr. J. Arnold Bargen, to conduct a clinical evaluation of the drug we now know as sulfasalazine in patients with ulcerative colitis. The study he performed was *double-blind, randomized, placebo-controlled,* and *prospective* in its design. When the data were analyzed and the drug was found to be effective, it was subsequently marketed in the United States and thereafter used throughout the world.

It is important to understand that sulfasalazine became available because a well-designed research project demonstrated its effectiveness. What made the clinical observations especially meaningful was that IBD patients participated in the required experimental studies and agreed to be evaluated periodically to assess the medication's effectiveness.

NEW DRUG DEVELOPMENT AND APPROVAL

A new drug becomes a marketable product and an acceptable therapy after a long and arduous process. First, the need for a new medication or a modification of an existing drug needs to be recognized and pharmaceutical firms staffed with research chemists must agree to undertake the laborious task of drug development. When it is developed, the proposed new drug must be shown in the laboratory to have the desired biological effect. The safety of the drug in varied doses then must be established in animals, followed by tests for safety in healthy human volunteers. Finally, a research project is designed to evaluate the new or modified drug in patients with a specific disease, IBD for example. The pharmaceutical company will recruit qualified clinical investigators, usually in major medical centers, who agree to enter their patients in the clinical study. Finally, the data obtained are analyzed statistically and a decision is reached regarding the drug's effectiveness.

When clinical testing is completed, a process that typically takes several years, the data are presented to the Food and Drug Administration (FDA) as part of a New Drug Application (NDA). The application is reviewed without bias, by experts who must decide if the drug is safe, whether it has been evaluated properly, and whether it will be effective in the specific disease for which approval is requested.

If procedures are followed properly, it is likely that the drug will be approved for use in humans. If steps were flawed in some way, studies may have to be repeated, more patients may have to be enrolled, or the study design may have to be modified to eliminate the possibility of reaching premature or invalid conclusions.

What are the important factors that reduce the likelihood that a clinical investigation will be flawed? You have already read the terms double-blind, randomized, placebo-controlled, and prospective. We will consider these terms in greater detail since they are central to a well designed clinical research project.

Because a clinical investigator believes the study drug should work, he/she may be prone to *investigator bias* in reporting clinical observations. Patients, too, may be biased (*patient bias*) because of what they may have read or heard about the drug's effects. To eliminate the possibility that these biases will occur, a clinical study should be double-blinded. A double-blind study is one in which neither the physician nor the patient knows whether the study drug is being administered, or whether the "drug" is actually a placebo. A placebo is a nondrug made to appear in every way like the test drug, but without its biological effects. In this way, response to the new drug can be measured against the effect of simply giving treatment. The drug is assigned a code number, known only to the pharmaceutical company's representative or a statistician who has assigned the number. In this way, both the objective evaluations of the physician and the subjective assessments of the patients are made blindly, without knowing whether the patient has received the drug or a placebo.

Many variables, such as age, sex, race, and duration and extent of illness, may influence the way a person responds to drugs when participating in a research project. Even the mere act of participating in a study, seeing the physician, keeping careful clinical records, and taking medications (even if only placebos) may make a difference in outcome and may complicate the interpretation of data. Up to 30% of patients entering clinical studies improve spontaneously without any therapy. This is known as the "placebo effect," which must be anticipated and incorporated in the study design before meaningful data can emerge.

To avoid bias in selecting which patients receive the actual drug or the placebo, study participants are *randomized*, or randomly assigned using a statistician's table of random numbers. This means that the true drug and the placebo might be administered to the first 10 people entering the study in no particular order. When large numbers of patients are enrolled in a study, half of the patients usually receive true drug and half receive placebo; they receive them in random order to ensure that the unknown variables have an equal chance of influencing a response to the true drug and the placebo.

In addition, a well designed clinical study should be *prospective* rather than retrospective. In a prospective study, data are gathered under controlled conditions from the beginning to the end of the study period. Such data are likely to be much more meaningful than retrospective data obtained from records of patients who received medications under uncontrolled conditions before the start of the study.

PARTICIPATING IN A CLINICAL STUDY

It is likely that someday you might be asked to participate in clinical research. Without your participation, meaningful research cannot take place and the development of drugs will be considerably retarded. Of course, you have the right to refuse participation at any time or to withdraw your participation once you have agreed to enter a study without worrying that your medical care will be jeopardized. Before participating in a study, you will be asked to sign an *informed consent*, which indicates that you understand the risks and benefits of the study, the alternatives in your treatment, and your option to withdraw from it at any time (*See Chapter 21*). If you or your physician feel that you are not doing well in the study, you may withdraw and continue treatment with conventional medications or surgery. In these instances, some patients have been found to have been receiving placebo and in others to be receiving the true drug.

Although the opportunity is not likely to arise that often, you have a responsibility to yourself and to other IBD patients to try to participate in well designed, meaningful clinical research whenever possible. Concerned investigators, courageous patients, and time are the key ingredients in a successful clinical study.

9 // Newer Medications

NEW SALICYLATE PREPARATIONS

Five aminosalicylic acid (5-ASA) is not really a new medication; it may be familiar to you as the active component of sulfasalazine (Azulfidine®). As you will remember from Chapter 4, sulfasalazine is composed of two compounds attached by a chemical bond, sulfapyridine and 5-ASA. The sulfapyridine and the bond protect 5-ASA and prevent it from being absorbed in the stomach and the upper small intestine before it reaches the inflamed colon. As sulfasalazine passes into the colon, the bacteria that normally live there break the chemical bond and release the two individual compounds. Most of the sulfapyridine is absorbed into the circulation, and is further broken down by the liver and eliminated through the kidneys. Most of the 5-ASA remains within the colon and is believed to have a topical antiinflammatory effect on the mucosal lining of the large intestine. Because the small intestine contains too few bacteria to split the bond, 5-ASA is not released from sulfasalazine before it reaches the colon.

With the knowledge that 5-ASA is the active ingredient in sulfasalazine, the pharmaceutical industry has developed new products that can deliver 5-ASA more precisely to the inflamed intestine with high doses of a relatively nontoxic, well-tolerated medication. The rationale for using 5-ASA as therapy for IBD is two-fold. First, many patients are unable to tolerate sulfasalazine in significant doses, either because of side effects that are dose-related (headache, dizziness, nausea, muscle aches) or because of allergic reactions (fevers, skin rashes, hemolytic anemia). Second, the amount of 5-ASA in the maximal tolerated dose of sulfasalazine may not be sufficient to heal active colitis in some individuals.

Since most of the side effects of sulfasalazine appear to be caused by sulfapyridine, it would be desirable to eliminate the sulfa portion altogether. Unfortunately, if 5-ASA alone is taken by mouth in an unprotected form, most of it dissolves and is absorbed quickly from the stomach or small intestine. To be effective, 5-ASA must either be delivered directly to the lower colon via an enema or suppository, or its oral form must be protected from absorption by coating it with a special substance or attaching it to a compound with few adverse side effects.

Recent studies have shown that 5-ASA enemas or suppositories are even more effective than oral sulfasalazine with or without the addition of steroids. Clinical researchers hope that by eliminating the side effects caused by sulfapyridine, 5-ASA can be delivered in even higher doses to the inflamed intestine. Because different preparations of 5-ASA are able to target the delivery of the drug to specific sites along the intestine, 5-ASA eventually will be used to treat disease of the small bowel as well as the colon.

5-ASA and 4-ASA Enemas and Suppositories

Enemas containing up to 4 gm (4000 mg) of active drug have undergone extensive study and appear to be quite safe when prepared in 60 to 100 ml of solution. The 5-ASA enema recently approved by the FDA is Rowasa® (Reid-Rowell). Enemas of this size can coat the lining of the colon all the way up the left side of the colon. Since disease is limited to the left colon in more than half of those with ulcerative colitis, most people should benefit from these enemas.

Five-ASA enemas appear to be a highly effective treatment for left-sided ulcerative colitis. Most patients with newly diagnosed ulcerative colitis will respond to this form of therapy, and even those whose symptoms have not responded to other treatments may do well with the 5-ASA enemas. However, some form of maintenance therapy, such as continued enema use, oral 5-ASA, or sulfasalazine, may be needed to prevent relapse. These enemas may also be useful in treating Crohn's disease of the lower colon, although this needs further study.

Users of 5-ASA enemas report a few side effects, including occasional abdominal cramps, headache, gas, nausea, and hair loss. However, one of the problems with using 5-ASA in an enema solution is the stability of the drug. 5-ASA is normally white or cream-colored and darkens to a brown color as the drug deteriorates. You should avoid using an enema product that has darkened in color, since we do not know the effects or safety of the breakdown products.

Suppositories containing 5-ASA are also being developed. A 500-mg suppository taken two or three times daily may be as effective as 5-ASA enemas for patients with ulcerative proctitis. It is possible that maintenance of remission can even be achieved with a single suppository taken each night. These products are also well tolerated and have few, if any, side effects.

Enemas of 4-ASA, a closely related compound used for many years in an oral form to treat tuberculosis, may also alleviate the symptoms of proctitis or left-sided ulcerative colitis. Although these enemas are still being developed, clinical studies have shown results similar to those of 5-ASA enemas.

Oral 5-ASA Products

Several different oral preparations of 5-ASA are currently under study and awaiting FDA approval. Among these, we probably have the most clinical information about olsalazine (Dipentum®, Pharmacia), a compound composed of two molecules of 5-ASA joined by the same chemical bond present in sulfasalazine. Like sulfasalazine, olsalazine passes through the stomach and small intestine and requires breakdown by colonic bacteria to release both molecules of 5-ASA. Olsalazine seems to be as effective as sulfasalazine in treating ulcerative colitis, and like all 5-ASA products lacks many of the side effects attributed to the sulfa portion of sulfasalazine. Some people taking high doses of olsalazine may develop diarrhea, but this is often overcome by taking small quantities at first, and then gradually increasing the dose or by reducing the dose. Because of the infrequency of major side effects, most people can tolerate higher total doses of 5-ASA than sulfsalazine.

Two other forms of oral 5-ASA are coated with acrylic resins in order to protect the drug from dissolution by stomach acid and allow it to be released further down the digestive tract. Asacol® (Norwich Eaton), which releases 400 mg of 5-ASA into the terminal ileum and colon, also seems to be as effective as sulfasalazine in treating and preventing relapses of ulcerative colitis. Studies of Asacol® in ileal and colonic Crohn's disease are currently underway. Salofalk® (SmithKline International) also uses an acrylic resin to deliver 5-ASA into the ileum and colon. Studies of Salofalk® for both ulcerative colitis and Crohn's disease of the ileum and colon seem promising, but it is questionable whether this drug will be marketed eventually in the United States.

In Pentasa® (Marion Laboratories), 5-ASA is protected within ethyl-cellulose beads. This preparation has been used in Europe for both ulcerative colitis and Crohn's disease, and also seems to be as effective as sulfasalazine in treating ulcerative colitis. Pentasa® capsules release the drug in a time-dependent manner; half the 5-ASA is released into the small intestine and the other half into the colon. In this preparation, more 5-ASA may be available higher up in the intestine than with other products, and Pentasa® may be a useful product for small bowel Crohn's disease as well as for colitis. Clinical studies examining a variety of dosing schedules are currently underway.

NEW IBD DRUGS ON THE HORIZON

One of the premises underlying medical research is that if we understand more about how a disease develops, we will be able to design and test better medical treatments for it. We have been most successful in treating those diseases whose cause and natural history we understand best. Unfortunately, since the cause of IBD is not yet known, our attempts to develop new drug treatments have been hampered. Hopefully, future research will reveal the cause of IBD and thus lay the foundation for specific therapy.

Many scientists think that IBD may be caused by an unidentified initiating event that attacks the body's immune response and ultimately results in what we recognize as IBD (*See Chapter 1*). Inflammation is a general term used to describe any disease process characterized by swelling, redness, and pain. Certain chemicals made by cells of the immune system mediate this inflammatory response and also promote the movement of white blood cells out of the bloodstream and into the intestinal tissue, thereby producing damage to the intestinal lining. Among these mediators are familiar compounds such as histamine, and others such as prostaglandins and leukotrienes.

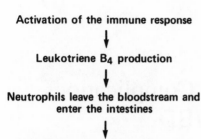

Activation of the immune response

↓

Leukotriene B₄ production

↓

Neutrophils leave the bloodstream and enter the intestines

↓

Neutrophils release compounds which are toxic for intestinal cells

FIG. 1. The role of leukotriene B_4 in IBD inflammation.

These compounds are important in many different inflammatory diseases besides IBD, including rheumatoid arthritis, asthma, and hay fever. The particular mediator for each disorder may help to determine therapy. Histamine plays an important role in hay fever and antihistamines are effective treatments. Prostaglandins aggravate arthritis, so aspirin and ibuprofen (Nuprin® or Advil®), which block prostaglandin production, are frequently beneficial. Because antihistamines, aspirin, and ibuprofen are not effective in treating IBD, we assume that histamine and prostaglandins are probably not of fundamental importance in the development of IBD. If we could identify the mediators of IBD, we would have a clue to help us develop specific therapy.

Whereas researchers are not certain which mediators are involved in IBD, there is some evidence that one group called the leukotrienes may be important. The most prominent leukotriene in IBD is leukotriene B_4, a compound that causes certain white blood cells, called neutrophils, to leave the blood stream and enter the intestinal tissue. Once in the inflamed tissue, the neutrophils release other compounds that may be toxic to the gut lining (Fig. 1). The concentration of leukotriene B_4 in the intestinal mucosa in IBD is at least 50 times greater than that in normal mucosa. There is also considerable evidence that the drugs currently used to treat IBD also affect leukotriene production.

White blood cells incubated in a test tube produce smaller amounts of leukotrienes if they are exposed to sulfasalazine, 5-aminosalicylic acid (5-ASA), or corticosteroids. Similarly, when patients with IBD are treated with sulfasalazine, 5-ASA, or corticosteroids, smaller amounts of leukotrienes are produced by their white blood cells than when no therapy is given; however, we do not know if this represents a direct inhibition of leukotriene production by these drugs or merely an indirect decrease in leukotriene production because of improvement in the bowel disease.

These studies of leukotriene B_4 have led to the possibility that IBD may be treated by blocking leukotriene B_4. A number of pharmaceutical companies have developed agents that block leukotriene production by white blood cells. Other pharmaceutical companies have drugs that prevent leukotrienes from interacting with neutrophils. Studies are underway to see if these drugs have the same effects when given to humans. If these studies are successful then we can expect that these drugs will be tested in IBD in the future.

10 / Managing the Complications of IBD

TREATMENT OF PERINEAL CROHN'S DISEASE

The development of perineal complications is one of the most distressing situations encountered by the person with Crohn's disease. The perineum is composed of the anal and genital areas and their surrounding tissues. This area, also called the perianal area, is affected in approximately 25% of patients with Crohn's disease. Perineal disease is more common when the large intestine is involved and is virtually always present in patients with Crohn's disease of the rectum.

Perineal complications include abscesses and fistulas, which drain pus or bowel contents into the skin or perforate into the vagina (in the female) or the scrotum (in the male). In addition, Crohn's disease may cause ulcerations that are slow to heal and new growths of tissue around the anal area, called skin tags, that are sometimes mistaken for hemorrhoids. Although some of these perineal complications are painless, abscesses can often be quite painful unless they drain spontaneously or are drained by surgical incision.

Perineal lesions may vary extensively in type and with the activity of the underlying bowel disease. Such variation in the expression of disease leads to different levels of treatment. Many simple perineal ulcers require no surgical treatment and will heal spontaneously as the disease is controlled medically. Surgical treatment of uncomplicated fistulas varies with the preference of the individual surgeon, many opting simply to open the fistulous tract. This is usually followed by slow but progressive healing. Others perform an operation in which some of the muscle fibers of the internal anal sphincter are divided in order to remove the origin of the fistula and achieve healing (*See Chapter 34*).

When an abscess occurs in the area around the anus, a surgical procedure is usually required to relieve pain and fever. As the operative wound heals, the fistula may remain but drainage from its opening usually gradually diminishes or disappears completely as the bowel disease improves. In addition, either metronidazole or 6-MP may be employed to encourage healing. (See a discussion of these medications in Chapters 6 and 7.) These medications are being used increasingly as alternatives to surgery or to reduce the extent of operation. Repetitive operations that sacrifice more and more of the muscular sphincters controlling the anus may lead to fecal incontinence. Whenever possible, those with perineal complications are encouraged to seek the care of colon and rectal surgeons who are experienced in handling these complications of Crohn's disease.

In rare instances, ulcerating and destructive lesions of the perineum may prove resistant to local measures and even to metronidazole or 6-MP therapy. Attempts to treat such lesions by leaving the rectum intact and diverting the flow of feces through a temporary ostomy are usually not successful. Surgical removal of the colon and rectum and creation of an ileostomy may be the only way to relieve the continued pain, social embarrassment, and interference with normal sexual function that these lesions may cause. After removal of the rectum and any contiguous disease, healing may occur more slowly than in patients afflicted with other problems requiring similar surgery. Patience and an experienced surgeon are usually the most important factors in the healing process.

TREATING THE ARTHRITIS OF IBD

In addition to the transient backaches and joint pains of normal life, there are several dozen diseases that are associated with more persistent and severe joint pain, often accompanied by signs of inflammation—redness, swelling, and warmth. Although patients with IBD may develop joint pains from any of these diseases, there are two types of arthritis that are particularly common in these patients.

Peripheral Arthritis

One type of arthritis, known as a peripheral arthritis, is characterized by pain, swelling, and stiffness in one or more of the joints of the arms and legs, such as the wrists, knees, and ankles. When untreated, the joints remain painful for several days to weeks, but unlike other forms of arthritis, there is no permanent damage. Once the inflammation disappears, the function of the joint returns to normal. This peripheral arthritis is more common in persons with colitis (Crohn's or ulcerative) and its severity usually parallels the degree of inflammation in the colon. Although we do not know the cause of this form of arthritis, it is believed that some of the inflammation represents an immunologic response to substances that may enter the body through the inflamed bowel wall.

Since patients with IBD can develop arthritis from a variety of conditions, accurate diagnosis is the first step in treatment. Although no laboratory test can definitively establish the diagnosis of peripheral arthritis of IBD, blood tests, joint fluid analysis, and x-rays of the joints are frequently needed to exclude other causes of joint pain.

Approaches to Treatment

Once the diagnosis of peripheral arthritis of IBD is established, there are three approaches to therapy. The first of these is appropriate rest of the inflamed joints combined with the use of splints and occasional moist heat. In order to prevent the inflamed joints from developing any limitation of motion and to loosen any tightened muscles, your physician may prescribe "range of motion" exercises, often with the help of a physical therapist. Heat is beneficial, whereas the application of ice packs to cool the joint is usually not recommended. In general, if a joint is red, warm, swollen, and tender, it needs rest more than exercise, whereas if it is primarily stiff, it needs exercise as well. It is only necessary to put a joint through a range of motion for 5 to 10 minutes a day to prevent muscle shortening and loss of movement.

The second approach to treatment consists of using medications, known as NSAIDs, which act in a manner similar to aspirin (Table 1). Because these medications may cause irritation of the stomach and aggravate the symptoms of IBD, they should be taken only with the close supervision of your physician. However, they are usually well tolerated and provide excellent reduction in the redness, swelling, and pain of inflamed joints. Occasionally, in persons who cannot tolerate these drugs, or whose arthritis does not respond to this treatment, low doses of steroids such as prednisone may be indicated. Steroids should be taken *only* when absolutely needed and then only in the lowest effective dose. When the arthritis involves a single joint, as frequently occurs in the peripheral arthritis of IBD, injection of steroids directly into the involved joint may provide rapid and effective reduction of symptoms.

The third approach to the treatment of this peripheral arthritis is to control the

TABLE 1. *Names of some nonsteroidal (nonaspirin) antiinflammatory drugs*

Generic name	Brand name
Indomethacin	Indocin®
Ibuprofen	Motrin®, Rufen®, Advil®, Nuprin®
Naproxen	Naprosyn®
Sulindac	Clinoril®
Piroxicam	Feldene®
Tolectin	Tolectin®
Meclofenamin acid*	Meclomen®
Phenylbutazone**	Butazolidin®
Ketoprofen	Orudis®
Diflunisal	Dolobid®
Choline salicylate	Trilisate®
Salsalate	Disalcid®
Fenoprofen	Nalfon®

*Frequently causes diarrhea and relatively contraindicated in IBD.
**High incidence of serious adverse drug reactions and should not be taken for more than 1 week.

colonic inflammation with the medications outlined in other parts of this book. Although total removal of the colon (colectomy) often permanently resolves the arthritis, colectomy is *never* recommended as primary therapy for joint pain alone because the arthritis of IBD is typically self-limiting and does not cause permanent joint damage.

Spinal Arthritis

Persons with IBD can also develop pain and stiffness in the joints of their spinal column. This arthritis of the spine is known as spondylitis. Persons with spondylitis, in contrast to those with peripheral arthritis, frequently have a special genetic marker known as the HLA B27 antigen. This same genetic marker is also found in patients with spondylitis from other causes and can be found by a blood test. Symptoms of spondylitis may precede the symptoms of IBD by months or even years, and the progression of the two conditions may not be parallel. Unlike the peripheral arthritis, in which irreversible changes do not occur, spondylitis *may* result in fusion (ankylosis) of the bones of the vertebral column leading to a permanent decrease in the range of motion of the back. The most frequent areas of involvement of the spine in patients with IBD are the sacroiliac joints, which are located on each side of the lowest portion of the spine where it joins to the pelvic bones. Pain and stiffness are frequently worse in the morning on arising and improve with activity. The restriction of rib motions may limit the ability to take a deep breath. In most cases, the active spondylitis of IBD rarely persists beyond age 40 years, although bony fusion and permanent disability may occur early in the course of illness.

The goal of therapy for spondylitis is to ensure maximum functional range of motion of the spine. This is accomplished by physical therapy using postural and stretching exercises (such as those illustrated in Figs. 1–7) in conjunction with the application of moist heat to the back. Moist heat reduces secondary muscle spasm, which in turn lessens pain and stiffness. Most patients also benefit from NSAIDs. Frequently these drugs must be taken for several years until all symptoms of back inflammation have disappeared. Steroids are usually contraindicated in treating spondylitis because of their tendency to produce a softening of the bones, called osteoporosis. Treatment of the intestinal inflammation usually has no effect on the course of spinal arthritis, and total colectomy is *not* recommended as a treatment for the spondylitis.

With proper treatment, most patients with arthritic symptoms from their IBD can be effectively treated to control their symptoms and remain free of functional disability.

SKIN COMPLICATIONS OF IBD

Skin complications occur with varying frequency in ulcerative colitis and Crohn's disease and, just as with joint and eye symptoms, are more common with

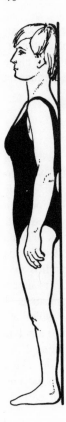

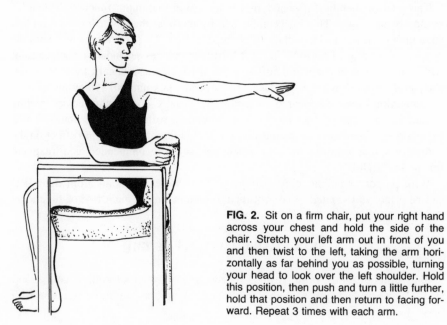

FIG. 1. Standing with your heels and seat against a wall and keeping your chin in, push your head back toward the wall and keep it back for the count of 5, then relax. Repeat 10 times.

FIG. 2. Sit on a firm chair, put your right hand across your chest and hold the side of the chair. Stretch your left arm out in front of you and then twist to the left, taking the arm horizontally as far behind you as possible, turning your head to look over the left shoulder. Hold this position, then push and turn a little further, hold that position and then return to facing forward. Repeat 3 times with each arm.

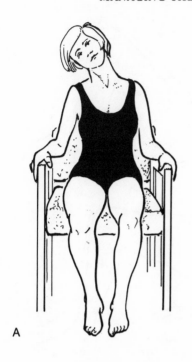

A

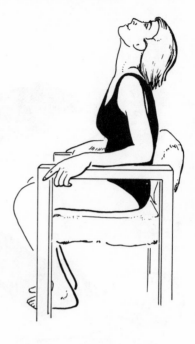

B

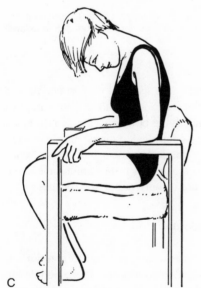

C

FIG. 3. A: Sit with your shoulders relaxed and chin drawn in, looking straight ahead. Bend your head sideways to bring your right ear toward your right shoulder, hold it there, make sure your shoulder muscles are still relaxed and bend a bit further, then return to straight. (As you do the side bending, the profile of your nose should remain in the same place, to make sure you don't turn your head.) Repeat to each side twice. **B:** Now tip your head back, looking up the wall and along the ceiling and bring it back to straight. Repeat. **C:** Change to tipping your head forward as far as possible to get your chin touching your neck, and return to straight with chin pulled in. Repeat.

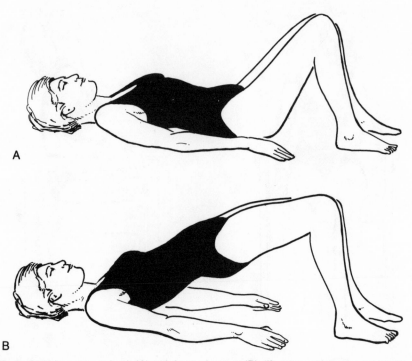

FIG. 4. Still lying on your back (**A**) with knees bent up (**B**), lift up your hips, so your seat is off the floor and there is a straight line from shoulder to knees. Hold for the count of 5, and lower. Repeat 5 times.

colonic than small bowel disease. These changes are seen not only in people with IBD but in those with other inflammatory diseases. Some of these skin complications are an indicator of the severity of the underlying bowel disease and disappear when bowel symptoms or disease activity is controlled. Others, like pyoderma gangrenosum, respond to local as well as systemic treatment but do not bear a close relationship to disease activity. Still others, such as rashes around the site of an ileostomy, need only local treatment and are of only minor significance.

Erythema Nodosum

Erythema nodosum is characterized by red, tender bumps on the anterior surface of the lower legs and occasionally on the thighs or arms. These nodules involve the lower subcutaneous layers of the skin and may be associated with fever and joint pains. The lesions resemble large, red insect bites but they may also appear as raised, red, diffusely sloping areas of skin rather than as separate nodules. Each individual nodule will usually persist for 3 to 6 weeks and may turn a darker color before it heals. The nodules do not usually ulcerate or form scars unless they

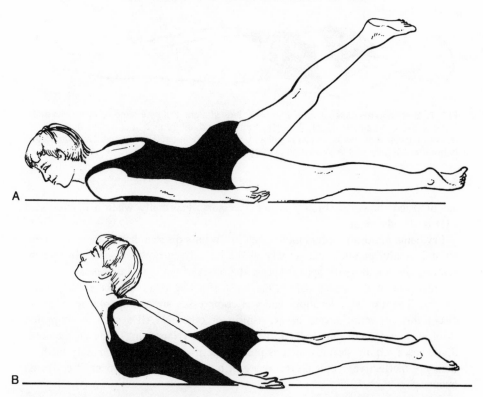

FIG. 5. Lie on your front, head turned to one side, hands by your sides. (If necessary, you may put a pillow under your chest, but not your waist, in order to get comfortable.) **A:** Raise one leg off the ground, keeping your knee straight, 5 times each leg, making sure your thigh comes off the ground. **B:** Raise your head and shoulders off the ground as high as you can 10 times.

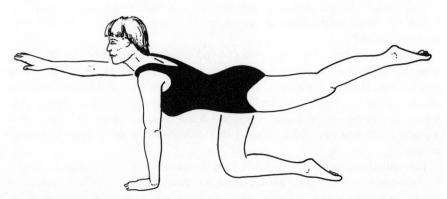

FIG. 6. Kneeling on the floor on all fours, stretch the opposite arm and leg out parallel with the floor and hold for the count of 10. Lower and then repeat with other arm and leg. Repeat 5 times each side.

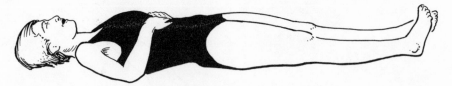

FIG. 7. Breathing exercises. Lie on your back, legs straight. Put your hands on your ribs at the sides of chest. Breathe in deeply through your nose and out through your mouth, pushing your ribs out against your hands as you breathe in. Repeat 10 times. (Remember, it is as important to breathe out fully as it is to breathe in deeply.)

are biopsied; however, biopsy is not necessary, especially when a diagnosis of IBD is already made.

Erythema nodosum occurs more often in Crohn's disease than in ulcerative colitis and usually parallels the activity of the underlying bowel disease. In rare instances, the nodules will appear before the onset of the bowel disease.

Treatment of the active IBD is the most effective treatment for erythema nodosum. Bed rest, leg elevation, and wet compresses are also helpful in relieving discomfort. In more severe cases, aspirin or other NSAIDs such as ibuprofen (Motrin®), indomethacin (Indocin®), or naproxen (Naprosyn®) may be required. Some cases require steroids such as prednisone if other antiinflammatory medications are ineffective. Topical creams are of no value in the treatment of erythema nodosum.

Pyoderma Gangrenosum

This severe skin problem is characterized by a painful area of deep undermining ulceration surrounded by irregular heaped-up borders. Pyoderma gangrenosum begins as groups of small pimples or pustules that coalesce, widen, and ulcerate. Although pyoderma occurs most commonly on the lower legs and feet, it may occur anywhere on the body.

There seems to be little correlation of pyoderma with the activity of the underlying bowel disease, which is usually ulcerative colitis. All ulcers of the skin in patients with IBD are not pyoderma and it is important that your physician evaluate any ulcers for other causes before therapy is begun. Although pyoderma gangrenosum may become secondarily infected and require treatment with antibiotics, it probably develops in IBD as a result of a disturbance in the immune regulatory system.

The initial treatment for pyoderma gangrenosum is usually local (topical) and the best results are obtained when lesions are treated early. Topical treatment of pyoderma gangrenosum includes silver nitrate applications and compresses of Burow's (aluminum acetate) or saline solution. Occasionally, steroid injections are given directly into the lesion itself or into the surrounding tissues. Steroids or drying agents such as benzoyl peroxide may also be applied directly to the ulcer. More difficult cases are treated with systemic steroids, antibiotics, dapsone (a sulfa drug), and occasionally with medications that alter the immune response (azathioprine or cyclophosphamide). Whereas surgery on the pyoderma lesion itself is occasionally required, colectomy does *not* necessarily control or improve this skin complication. The decision about whether colectomy is advisable should be based solely on the activity of the bowel disease and its response to medical therapy.

Aphthous Stomatitis (Mouth Ulcers)

Aphthous ulcers are small mouth sores that may appear in as many as 10% of IBD patients. As with other extraintestinal problems in IBD, these lesions are often a sign that bowel symptoms are active; in rare cases, these oral ulcers may be the first sign of IBD.

These aphthous ulcers appear as single or multiple shallow erosions in the inner surface of the mouth, including the tongue and the hard and soft palate. They are often quite painful and may interfere with eating and talking for as long as 1 to 2 weeks. Fortunately, they heal without scarring.

Local remedies may provide short-term relief. A liquid formula of tetracycline swished in the mouth for 2 to 3 minutes will reduce the duration, size, and pain of these lesions. Topical steroids in a special oral preparation are sometimes helpful, but need to be applied 4 to 6 times daily. Steroid sprays are also beneficial. Topical anesthetic agents like lidocaine will help relieve pain until the mouth sores disappear when bowel symptoms subside or are controlled with medications.

Rashes at the Ostomy Site

Rashes and skin irritations can appear at and around ileostomy and colostomy sites. These rashes typically appear as red small bumps and occasionally even small blisters. This type of local skin irritation is called eczematous or irritant dermatitis and is caused by skin contact with the bowel contents or by allergic sensitivity to the ostomy appliance or its adhesive. Bacteria or yeast from the bowel may secondarily irritate the skin around the stoma.

These irritations should be treated promptly to prevent skin erosions or peristomal ulcers. Once the cause of the irritation has been determined, treatment should be started. Topical steroids are helpful to ease simple irritation. Treatment with karaya gum or cholestyramine (Questran®) in an ointment base has also been used for peristomal irritation. Occasionally, a protective covering or skin barrier is necessary. There are many ointments and biological synthetic dressings that provide reasonable protection from further damage by these irritants. If a bacterial or fungal cause is found, then oral antibiotics or special topical creams may be needed to clear these infections.

In general, the best protection against these rashes is meticulous care of the ostomy site. It is extremely important to develop a regular regimen of changing the ostomy bag and keeping the skin around the stoma clean and dry. The ostomy appliance should fit snugly around the stoma to prevent leakage of bowel contents onto the exposed skin. Today, many types of appliances and adhesives are available so that most of these skin problems can be avoided.

Perineal Irritations

A variety of skin problems may occur in the area surrounding the rectum in patients with IBD. These problems occur almost exclusively with Crohn's disease and include fissures, fistulas, and abscesses. There is a complete discussion of the surgical treatment of perineal complications in Chapter 34.

EYE PROBLEMS IN IBD

The most common type of eye inflammation associated with IBD is uveitis, or inflammation of the uveal tract. The uvea is the middle layer of the eye wall that contains many of the blood vessels nourishing the eye. Since the uvea borders many important parts of the eye, inflammation of this layer can affect the adjacent cornea, retina, sclera, and other vital parts of the eye. Fortunately, only a few IBD patients ever develop uveitis, and proper diagnosis and prompt treatment may prevent possible loss of vision. Other ocular problems occur less commonly and therefore will not be discussed here. For completeness, however, they include inflammation of the surface of the eye (conjunctivitis, episcleritis), back of the eye (retinitis), and optic nerve (optic neuritis).

Symptoms of Uveitis

Uveitis causes sensitivity to light (photophobia), blurred vision, pain, and redness of the eye. Symptoms may come on suddenly or slowly with just gradual blurring of vision. When the uvea is inflamed near the front of the eye and the iris (colored part of the eye) is involved, this is called iritis. If the uvea is inflamed in the middle of the eye involving the ciliary body, this condition is called cyclitis. Iridocyclitis inflames both the iris and ciliary body, and is the most common form of uveitis of IBD. Iridocyclitis generally involves both eyes and, just as with the other extraintestinal manifestations in IBD, is usually seen in patients with colonic disease. Iridocyclitis tends to be recurrent and does not closely parallel bowel disease activity. Uveitis may occur in up to 12% of individuals with ulcerative colitis. It is much more common with accompanying spinal arthritis, where it affects up to 50% of patients. Uveitis occurs less often in Crohn's disease and may involve 10% of patients.

Diagnosis of Uveitis

Anyone with IBD should visit an eye specialist regularly and certainly when symptoms such as pain, redness, or blurred vision occur. An ophthalmologist will use special instruments such as a slit lamp to examine the inside of the eye and can often make a specific diagnosis and recommend therapy at the time of the examination. Uveitis may resemble other common eye irritations, such as conjunctivitis (Fig. 8). Typically in uveitis, however, redness encircles the cornea and its intensity increases as it approaches the central part of the eye (Fig. 9); in conjunctivitis, the pattern is reversed and the most severe inflammation is seen around the edges of the eye.

Treatment of Uveitis

The uveitis associated with IBD usually responds to treatment with eye drops containing steroids and pupil dilators that reduce inflammation and relieve pain. However, unless your underlying bowel disease is treated successfully, you will probably develop recurrent bouts of eye inflammation. Removal of the diseased colon (colectomy) sometimes diminishes the severity of uveitis but rarely prevents its recurrence altogether.

If any type of uveitis is left untreated, it may lead to complications such as high intraocular pressure (glaucoma), clouding of the lens (cataracts), or new blood

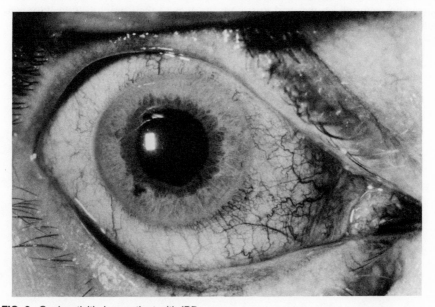

FIG. 8. Conjunctivitis in a patient with IBD.

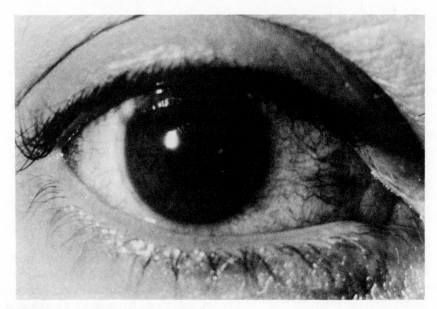

FIG. 9. Uveitis complicating IBD.

vessel formation (neovascularization). If these complications are advanced, conventional eye surgery or laser surgery may be necessary. Proper diagnosis and prompt treatment of uveitis are essential to prevent the development of these sight-threatening complications, and to restore the eyes to their previously healthy condition.

11// Treating Psychological Problems Caused by IBD

Psychological problems are common among the general population. For example, approximately 1 out of every 7 Americans has some anxiety disorder and 1 out of 12 will experience a major depression at some point in his/her life. Although the frequency of psychological problems in people with IBD is not known, common sense suggests that the added burdens these chronic illnesses place on people's lives would make these problems even more common than they are in the general population. Many factors such as age of onset, severity and length of illness, as well as a person's basic personality influence the impact of IBD. Thus IBD can be only a minor nuisance or it can dominate every aspect of life. This chapter will describe the more common psychological problems that IBD can produce.

DEPRESSION

Depression is the most common psychological problem caused by IBD. Although many people with Crohn's disease or ulcerative colitis occasionally feel "blue" or "down" for several hours or days, a major or severe depression should be viewed as an illness and may have both mental and physical effects. Common symptoms that may occur alone or in combination are extreme tiredness, insomnia (or the opposite—excessive need for sleep), loss of appetite with weight loss (or its opposite—overeating), difficulty in concentrating, crying spells and, at times, wishes to die or even kill oneself.

IBD can trigger a major depression in many ways. This occurs most commonly when your illness is "out of control" or when it forces you to curtail normal activities like work, school, or social life. Depression may also increase the way you perceive pain, setting up cycles in which sickness and pain create depression, which may increase feelings of sickness and more pain. Also, you should keep in mind that corticosteroids such as prednisone can cause or aggravate depression.

On the positive side, major depression is almost always treatable. After a careful assessment of the contributing factors, a psychiatrist or psychologist puts together an individualized treatment program. Such a plan is usually worked out in cooperative fashion between you, the physicians involved in your care, and the therapist. This plan may include your IBD medications (including lowering of steroids if possible), using antidepressants, and individual counseling or psychotherapy. At times, family therapy or group therapy with other IBD patients is extremely valuable and helps the patient develop a support system (*See Chapter 16*). With such a treatment program, most depressions begin to improve within 2 to 3 weeks and may resolve in 2 to 4 months. Depressions may recur, however, and may need further treatment.

ANXIETY

Anxiety is probably the second most common psychological problem affecting people with IBD. There are many day-to-day anxieties for a person with chronic bowel disease: Will I find a bathroom in time? Will I have a lot of pain today? What should I eat? It is also understandable to be concerned about the long-term outcome of IBD, especially when confronting fears about cancer or an ostomy. Although most people with IBD are able to control their fears and concerns, at times anxiety levels may escalate and cause physical symptoms such as insomnia, palpitations, shortness of breath, and diarrhea. There are some people whose IBD actually worsens under the stress of worry.

Fortunately, anxiety disorders, like depression, are generally treatable. After making sure that other medical conditions, such as thyroid disease, or drugs such as prednisone are not causing the anxiety symptoms, your psychotherapist will develop a plan with you to decrease or remove specific stresses. Part of this plan may include learning new coping skills and taking tranquilizers. If there is any evidence that your IBD is being made worse by stress, a plan of this sort should be started even if anxiety is not a severe problem. To find out if stress or other emotional factors are playing a role, it's a good idea to keep a diary for at least 2 to 3 weeks in which you chart daily events, emotional reactions to these events, and your bowel symptoms. This diary can be reviewed by the "team" to see if there are any relationships between life stresses, social issues, emotional factors, and bowel symptoms.

DENIAL OF ILLNESS

For some people, IBD is a very difficult illness to accept. Particularly difficult may be a specific aspect of IBD, such as its lifelong course, the unpredictability of relapses, or the possibility of an ostomy or cancer.

To cope with this problem, some people deny in whole, or in part, that they "really" have IBD. As an expression of this denial, they may fail to take medications regularly or may eat foods that they know will worsen their bowel disease. Occasionally, some individuals may stop taking medications altogether, avoid seeing the physician, or deny that they are having a relapse until they are seriously ill and need to be hospitalized. Understandably, denial is most common among people in their teens and twenties, largely because their illness robs them of some control over their lives—especially their social lives. Young people need to be accepted by their peers and having a chronic bowel disease can interfere with that process. Young people may consider IBD a weakness or a threat to their attractiveness.

The starting point in helping most people accept a chronic illness and its proper treatment is to help them to understand how unproductive and dangerous denial is. An understanding therapist can help an individual discover what it is about having IBD that makes it so difficult to accept. Mutual help groups and support groups, such as the ones conducted by chapters of the Crohn's & Colitis Foundation of America, are extremely helpful in encouraging people with IBD and their family members to share coping strategies and to provide support for each other. Chapter 17 contains a full discussion of these groups and what they can offer.

12 // Treatment of Children with IBD

Young people with IBD experience the same psychosocial pressures and expectations as all children and adolescents. Therefore, any approach to treating IBD in these young people should consider that they must simultaneously negotiate this difficult transition to adulthood and, in addition, deal with a disease that causes them pain, embarrassment, and social isolation. For example, one important task of adolescence is to separate from one's parents while achieving independence. Chronic illness, with its need for regular visits to the doctor and chronic use of medications, fosters dependency and presents obstacles to this growth process. Furthermore, although healthy teenagers work full time to conform in behavior, dress, and appearance, young people with IBD are often faced with unpredictable bowel patterns, having to find a bathroom without friends knowing, and dealing with troublesome changes in appearance caused by medications.

Another important milestone of puberty is a marked growth spurt. Physical growth and development are measured in weight gain, height increase, and sexual maturation, all of which are closely related. While the teenage girl expects dramatic changes in her body and regularly checks for breast development, the teenage boy may compare his pubic hair and genital development with that of his friends. Unfortunately, children with IBD, particularly Crohn's disease, may experience a delay in growth and sexual maturation; this may cause them to feel a lack of self-esteem when they compare their physical changes with those of their peers.

THE IMPORTANCE OF NUTRITION

How IBD causes growth failure is unclear, but there is no doubt that inadequate caloric intake plays a major role. Healthy adolescents moving through puberty usually require about 30 calories per pound of body weight each day to achieve their ultimate height potential. On the other hand, the youngster with active IBD (especially if there has been weight loss or inadequate weight gain) requires up to 45 calories per pound of body weight each day for normal growth. Intake of these vital calories is made more difficult by the poor appetite and abdominal pain associated with eating that patients with IBD experience.

There are several approaches that can be used in the home to provide extra calories for these young people. Oral nutritional supplements are sometimes helpful but are usually poorly tolerated over long periods of time. Children may complain bitterly of the taste and often cannot tolerate the large volumes necessary to achieve the numbers of calories needed for growth.

To deal with these issues, teenagers have been encouraged to pass their own nasogastric tubes at night, allowing the infusion of nutritional supplements continuously during sleep. With this approach, an additional 1500 calories per 24 hours can be provided. Young people receiving this treatment have experienced significant increases in weight and height. Obviously, using tube feedings takes motivation on the part of the youngster and continuous support by the family and the physician or nurse. The fact that the tube is removed each morning is a strong motivating factor, since it allows the student to attend school and perhaps participate in the usual daily activities. Tube feedings can also be discontinued if necessary on weekends and vacations, or if the child goes to summer camp. In this case, the camp personnel should be alerted so they may provide an adequate diet with supplemental calories. Caloric requirements in children with IBD may be even greater during the summer months because of increased physical exercise.

Intravenous nutrients may also be infused at home through a "central line" during sleeping hours. A special type of catheter is inserted surgically into a large vein in the neck or near the shoulder. This procedure is performed in the hospital with local anesthesia. Once inserted, the catheter can remain in the body for extended periods of time, allowing the nightly infusions of high caloric solutions. The central line is capped during the day, allowing attendance at school. This approach entails more risks than tube feedings, mainly because of the potential for infection at the catheter site. Meticulous hygiene and regular cleansing of the site can minimize the risk of infection.

MEDICATIONS

The medications that are prescribed for children and adolescents with IBD are the same as those prescribed for adults. Sometimes there is disagreement about what doses of medications a child with IBD needs to avoid adverse side effects. Since medication dosages are essentially based on their use in adults rather than in children, much more research needs to be done on the unique requirements of the child who needs medical treatment for IBD.

Sulfasalazine (Azulfidine®)

For the child with active disease, most pediatric gastroenterologists prescribe sulfasalazine in a daily dose of 30 to 40 mg/pound of the child's body weight, divided in 2 to 4 doses. Therefore, a 100-pound child would receive the adult dose of 3 to 4 gm or 6 to 8 tablets (500 mg/tab) each day. After an adequate response, the dosage could be decreased to about 15 mg/pound per day, the equivalent of 1.5 gm or 3 tablets. To avoid embarrassment, children should not be expected to take medication in school. It is preferable that they take their pills in the morning and evening with meals and possibly before bedtime. Liquid sulfasalazine (250 mg/5 cc) is available for young children or for those unable or unwilling to swallow tablets. It may be easier to crush the tablets than to refill the liquid prescription constantly and to keep multiple bottles in the house. Except for allergic reactions resulting from the sulfa part of this medication, there are few serious side effects observed with these dosages. Sulfasalazine therapy sometimes causes the urine to appear dark or orange colored. This is to be expected and should not be mistaken for blood in the urine. Occasionally, youngsters will complain of nausea, headaches, and dizziness, which tend to disappear over time or when the dosage of medication is reduced. Although there is an aspirin-like component (5-ASA) in sulfasalazine, platelet and blood clotting functions (which are impaired by regular aspirin) remain normal.

Sulfasalazine is a medication that is taken for long periods of time without any serious consequences from its chronic use. Studies have indicated that the sulfa in sulfasalazine does not cause injury to the kidneys of children who have been on this medication for 1 to 2 years.

Corticosteroids (Prednisone, Medrol®, Hydrocortisone)

Corticosteroids may be given rectally, orally, or intravenously. The route of administration depends on which areas of intestine are involved and on the severity of disease (*See Chapter 5*). When IBD involves the rectum or the rectum and lower colon, and the child is having frequent bloody stools accompanied by urgency, rectal steroids are commonly prescribed either as an enema or in a foam. A small amount of the steroids given rectally is absorbed into the bloodstream and may cause cosmetic side effects and even growth suppression, although less commonly than with oral steroids. Rectal preparations may be used together with oral or intravenous steroids. This is done in an attempt to deliver a higher dose of medication to the inflamed colon or to try and lower the total dose of absorbed steroids, thereby diminishing any adverse side effects.

Having to take medicine rectally is particularly disturbing and embarrassing to the child or adolescent. You should be ready to offer help in administering these rectal medications but be prepared to withdraw if your help is rejected.

Side Effects of Corticosteroids

The cosmetic side effects of steroids are quite disturbing and may lead to poor compliance in children and adolescents. Acne and excessive growth of facial and body hair are transient and disappear when the dosage is lowered or the medication is discontinued. Stretch marks may occasionally result from steroid treatment and be permanent. These stretch marks typically lighten in color with time but do not disappear. Fortunately, children do not usually develop this problem. Steroids cause edema and with prolonged use result in weight gain and swelling of the body. Particularly disturbing is the so-called "moon face." Reducing the salt intake can diminish this effect but will not prevent or cure it. Salt should not be added to the diet, and foods and beverages high in salt content, such as potato chips, ham, pickles, etc., should be avoided. On the other hand, a "no salt" or very low salt diet is unpalatable, not necessary, and may result in diminished caloric intake. Discussing ways to reduce unnecessary salt with a nutritionist is helpful.

There are many risks of long-term steroid use in adults (*See Chapter 5*). In children, however, cosmetic changes and growth suppression are the only two problems that occur with any regularity and both are dose-related. Steroids suppress growth by interfering with bone growth. Uncontrolled disease activity also significantly inhibits growth and development. It is the task of the physician to balance the risks of steroids against their benefits in reducing disease activity. If disease activity can be controlled by using steroids on alternate days rather than daily, growth retardation may be minimized.

There is no evidence that the child or adolescent taking steroids is more susceptible to colds or other infections. One exception to this is the risk of overwhelming chicken pox infection. Any child on steroids who is exposed to chicken pox should receive an injection of zoster hyperimmune globulin. This injection provides antibodies to limit the severity of the disease. It is very important that the child on corticosteroids be followed closely for any complication after such an exposure or during the period of illness.

When steroids are administered as medication, they suppress the normal output of steroids by the adrenal gland. Such a "sleeping" adrenal gland may not respond to stress, such as surgery or severe infection, in the appropriate fashion. Thus, it is recommended that children who have received high doses or continuous steroids during the preceding 12 to 18 months and who are undergoing surgery be given additional steroids for the procedure itself and in the subsequent 24 to 48 hours.

There is no doubt that steroid therapy carries with it certain risks, but there is also little doubt that steroids are a vital medical therapy for the health and well-being of children with IBD. In each case, the benefits of steroid therapy must be balanced against its risks.

Metronidazole (Flagyl®)

Metronidazole is used in children and adolescents with perianal Crohn's disease and as an alternative to sulfasalazine and perhaps steroids for Crohn's disease of the colon. The dosage prescribed depends on the weight of the child (5 to 10 mg/pound/day) and is conveniently given with meals. Teenagers should be told that alcohol and metronidazole do not mix and may result in severe nausea and vomiting.

Most children who take metronidazole for many months begin to experience a feeling of "pins and needles" in their hands or feet. Some even complain of losing all feeling in their extremities and of being extremely sensitive to cold. When metronidazole is discontinued, this complication will diminish and subsequently disappear, although total relief may take weeks to months.

13 // Pregnancy and IBD

Since Crohn's disease and ulcerative colitis are illnesses that occur during the childbearing years, many questions are likely to arise concerning fertility, the use of IBD medications before conception, and the safety of medical and surgical treatment in the pregnant woman with IBD. This chapter will address these important questions.

FERTILITY IN WOMEN

Although women with IBD are often concerned that their disease will interfere with conception, evidence suggests that ulcerative colitis, whether active or inactive, does *not* reduce fertility. However, women with Crohn's disease may be less able to conceive, especially if their disease is active. In Crohn's disease, the ovaries and fallopian tubes, especially on the right side of the abdomen, may not function normally because of their proximity to inflamed bowel. In addition, the tendency of the disease to cause fistulas and abscesses in the vaginal or rectal areas may cause pain and thus interfere with intercourse. Fertility can usually be restored to normal when the symptoms of active Crohn's disease are brought under control with medical treatment.

A major factor leading to a reluctance to become pregnant is the fear that the disease might worsen during pregnancy or the fetus might be abnormal as a result of the disease. Despite this fear, most women with IBD are eventually able to conceive and give birth to normal healthy babies. Gastroenterologists often advise their patients to wait until they are in remission before attempting to conceive.

FERTILITY IN MEN

Infertility in men with IBD may be caused by severe disease or treatment with sulfasalazine. Within 2 months of starting the drug, the semen may become less dense and the sperm abnormal and less motile. Although some degree of semen abnormality has been observed in 86% of men taking sulfasalazine, this does not necessarily prevent impregnation. Moreover, these abnormalities are reversible when the drug is stopped. Semen quality begins to improve within 2 months after the drug is discontinued. The patient may have a hard time deciding whether to risk the consequences of stopping sulfasalazine to allow impregnation. Since the damage to sperm is caused by the sulfapyridine component, and not the 5-ASA component of sulfasalazine, the new salicylate preparations awaiting FDA approval may solve this problem without the risk of aggravating the disease.

Another cause for compromised fertility in the male with IBD may be the inability to have an adequate erection or ejaculation as a result of surgery to remove the rectum (as in proctocolectomy with ileostomy). This has been a greater concern in patients with ulcerative colitis where the rectum is removed than in Crohn's disease where it is often used for anastomosis. The newer operations for ulcerative colitis that preserve the rectum (ileoanal anastomosis) make this unusual complication even rarer.

HOW IBD MEDICATIONS AFFECT PREGNANCY

You may get conflicting opinions about whether you should start or even continue your IBD medications during pregnancy. In general, obstetricians prefer that all medications be stopped during pregnancy, while gastroenterologists favor continuing them to control disease activity. Since about 85% of all patients with ulcerative colitis or Crohn's disease are taking either sulfasalazine, steroids, or other medications at any given time, this is an issue that is likely to be encountered during pregnancy.

The obstetrician is naturally concerned about the safety of the fetus and may worry that these drugs will cause prematurity, low birth weight, stillbirth, spontaneous abortion, or genetic abnormalities. As you might imagine, the gastroenterologist must balance these concerns against his/her own concerns that IBD symptoms will worsen and cause harm to both mother and fetus. The following material summarizes what is currently known about the toxicity during pregnancy of the drugs used most commonly in the treatment of IBD.

Sulfasalazine

There is theoretical concern that sulfasalazine can cause fetal jaundice because other sulfa drugs do. However, this has never been reported and the risk must be very small indeed. The drug does cross the placenta to the fetus, and it also is expressed with the breast milk. Although some studies have shown that the amount of sulfasalazine or its components that reaches the nursing infant is small, most physicians recommend that women with IBD who need to take sulfasalazine not attempt to nurse their infants.

Sulfasalazine may impair the absorption of folic acid, a vitamin that is important to fetal development. Folate deficiency, especially in the early weeks of pregnancy, may cause defective cell formation, impaired cell growth, and damage to the placenta which, in turn, could lead to spontaneous abortion or congenital anomalies. If you are taking sulfasalazine while pregnant, your obstetrician or gastroenterologist will probably recommend that you take folic acid supplements to correct any possible deficiency of this vitamin.

Corticosteroids

Whereas steroids can increase the rates of abortion, stillbirths, and congenital anomalies in animals, prematurity, stillbirths, cleft palate and other congenital malformations occur rarely in humans. Breastfeeding while on steroids appears to be safe, and they may be taken when needed for an acute flare-up of IBD. Just as in the nonpregnant patient with IBD, they should be tapered and discontinued as soon as possible. Experience with this approach suggests that risk to the fetus is minimal.

Metronidazole and Other Antibiotics

Metronidazole has been shown to cause genetic mutations in bacteria and genetic changes and tumors in laboratory animals (*See Chapter 6*). In a study of more than 3000 pregnant women treated with short-term metronidazole for vaginal infections, no increase in congenital anomalies was found. The absolute safety of this drug in pregnancy is not established, however, and use of metronidazole should be avoided (if possible) during the early months. The drug is also not recommended in nursing mothers because it is excreted in the breast milk and we do not know its long-term effects on newborn infants.

We do not know enough about the effects of other antibiotics given during pregnancy, and in general, it is better to avoid them unless absolutely necessary. It is known that tetracycline taken by pregnant women may cause damage to the bones and teeth of the fetus. Probably all antibiotics are excreted in breast milk and therefore the same concerns apply about their use during nursing as about their use during pregnancy.

Immunosuppressive Agents: 6-MP and Azathioprine

There have been rare reports of congenital abnormalities in humans taking these agents during pregnancy, although normal infants have been born to patients with acute and chronic leukemias, lupus nephritis, and kidney transplants who have been treated with large doses of these and other immunosuppressive drugs during pregnancy. Healthy pregnancies in IBD patients treated with immunosuppressives have also been reported. In these cases, women taking 6-MP who became pregnant against the advice of their physicians chose not to have therapeutic abortions and proceeded to deliver normal infants. Nevertheless, most gastroenterologists are concerned about the possible genetic effects on future offspring of women taking immunosuppressives during pregnancy. There is less concern about using these drugs during the second and third trimesters than during the first. If a woman taking 6-MP or azathioprine decides that she wishes to become pregnant, it is recommended that the drug be stopped 2 to 3 months before planning conception, if possible.

There is no available information about the effects of 6-MP or azathioprine on a pregnancy when these drugs are taken by the father. However, it is prudent to stop them before planning a pregnancy.

HOW DOES IBD INFLUENCE THE PREGNANCY?

A recent study examined the outcome of 147 pregnancies in women with Crohn's disease or ulcerative colitis. Overall, the incidence of prematurity, stillbirths, and developmental defects was no greater in these women than in the general population. However, the incidence of spontaneous abortion was 12.2%, slightly higher than normal. The number of premature births and spontaneous abortions was considerably higher in those receiving treatment compared with those who were untreated. This trend was particularly evident in the Crohn's disease patients. Although fetal complications were more common in women who were treated during their pregnancy, the incidence of these complications was even greater when the disease was *active* during pregnancy, regardless of whether or not those patients received drug treatment.

The adverse effect of disease activity on the fetus was more apparent in Crohn's disease than in ulcerative colitis. The more devastating effect of disease activity than drug therapy on fetal outcome supports the use of IBD medications during pregnancy when there is *any* indication of active disease. This does not include therapy with immunosuppressives, however, for the reasons already discussed.

DOES PREGNANCY INFLUENCE THE COURSE OF IBD?

Available studies of large numbers of IBD patients indicate that when IBD is inactive at the time of conception, it is likely to remain inactive throughout the pregnancy. Active disease at the beginning of pregnancy is likely to persist and may worsen as the pregnancy progresses. Exacerbations of ulcerative colitis are most likely to occur during the first trimester of pregnancy, while Crohn's disease is more likely to become active during the third trimester. There is no evidence to suggest that IBD diagnosed for the first time during pregnancy will be any more severe than at other times.

In the past, therapeutic abortion was commonly employed in pregnant women with IBD because physicians anticipated a remission of disease when the pregnancy was terminated. However, experience accumulated over many years has shown that therapeutic abortion has *not* served to reverse the course of either ulcerative colitis or Crohn's disease, and should not be performed solely for that purpose.

Another area of concern has been the possibility that IBD will recur in the post-partum period. According to older studies, exacerbations of ulcerative colitis occasionally occurred postpartum, attributable to rapid hormonal changes immediately after delivery.

In Crohn's disease, the postpartum exacerbation was so commonplace that recommendations to administer ACTH, in an almost prophylactic fashion, were often made. More recent studies suggest that the postpartum period is really a continuation of the third trimester of pregnancy, and that if disease is active late in pregnancy, it will continue to be active and possibly even worsen during the postpartum period.

In short, the outlook for women with ulcerative colitis or Crohn's disease is the same regardless of whether or not they are pregnant, and the activity of IBD during any one pregnancy is of no predictive value for future pregnancies.

DIAGNOSTIC PROCEDURES DURING PREGNANCY

The use of x-rays should be avoided throughout pregnancy even though the risk to the fetus is present probably only in the first trimester. If needed to assess disease activity or to plan a change in therapy, rigid or flexible sigmoidoscopy with biopsies can be performed at any time during pregnancy, as can limited colonoscopy and upper gastrointestinal endoscopy. A full colonoscopy is technically more demanding during pregnancy and probably carries a greater risk. Nonetheless, it can be performed if indicated.

HOW SHOULD IBD BE TREATED DURING PREGNANCY?

Sulfasalazine has been shown to be effective in treating and preventing relapses of ulcerative colitis and might have similar effects in some cases of Crohn's disease. Therefore, if this drug is part of your treatment plan and if you are in remission, it probably should be continued throughout pregnancy and the postpartum period. If you have not been taking sulfasalazine and your disease becomes active, the pregnancy should not discourage you and your doctor from using the drug.

Steroids should be reduced gradually and stopped before or during pregnancy unless they are needed to control disease activity. Steroids can be started or reintroduced at any time during the pregnancy if IBD worsens. The course of your pregnancy is likely to be smoother when your disease is brought into remission, even by using steroids, than if you are pregnant in the presence of active disease.

Immunosuppressive drugs and metronidazole should not be introduced during pregnancy since many questions about possible fetal damage still remain unanswered. For the same reason, pregnancy should be postponed while you are on these drugs. If pregnancy does occur while on 6-MP or azathioprine, therapeutic abortion is recommended. However, there have been no instances of fetal damage in those few women taking 6-MP who chose to continue their pregnancy despite this advice.

Nonspecific antidiarrheal agents such as Imodium® and Lomotil®, and narcotics such as DTO should be used with caution, as they should be at any other time. This is particularly important in order to avoid respiratory depression and possible addiction in the newborn.

If you have active Crohn's disease and have not been able to conceive, your physician should continue treatment until your disease is brought into remission. If you cannot become pregnant at that point, it is reasonable to pursue a fertility evaluation.

The outlook for the pregnant woman with IBD and the survival and good health of her fetus correlate best with inactivity of the disease. Therefore, patient and physician should agree on a treatment plan to bring the disease into remission, if possible, before planning a pregnancy. If IBD becomes active during pregnancy, you need not be reluctant to use appropriate medical therapy to bring it into remission.

14 / IBD in Older People

Before beginning treatment, it is extremely important for the gastroenterologist to distinguish between older persons in whom the disease began when they were considerably younger, and those with recent onset of symptoms. The diagnosis of new IBD in the elderly must be made with caution and skepticism, since only 20% of patients with IBD can be expected to develop the disease in later life. In fact, most instances of new onset colitis in people beyond 60 years of age are not true IBD, but rather colitis caused by infections, reduced blood flow (ischemia), systemic disorders, or medications. Each of these types of colitis requires a different form of treatment.

The medical therapy of ulcerative colitis or Crohn's disease in the older person is quite similar to the treatment of these diseases in younger individuals. However, many physicians are reluctant to use moderate to high doses of corticosteroids, such as prednisone, for prolonged periods in the elderly because of a higher incidence of undesirable side effects.

The side effects include salt and water retention (with a resulting increase in blood pressure, swelling of the ankles, and shortness of breath in patients with preexisting heart disease), reduction of the potassium level in the blood (especially in persons taking diuretics), weakness, osteoporosis, infections (especially vaginal yeast infections), cataracts, and glaucoma. Despite this frightening menu of side effects, prednisone can be a lifesaving medication, and poses little risk in the short-term management of the sick patient. Indeed, it is still the most valuable medication in the treatment of severe colitis and Crohn's disease. All older patients on continuous prednisone therapy should have periodic check-ups with an internist and an ophthalmologist.

It is advisable to supplement long-term sulfasalazine therapy in the elderly patient with the vitamin folic acid, because sulfasalazine interferes with the intestinal absorption of dietary folate. Folic acid is important in the synthesis of protein and red blood cells and absorption of dietary folate may also be reduced with aging. Although there are no scientific studies specifically supporting this recommendation, many physicians use supplemental folic acid in patients receiving long-term sulfasalazine.

Surgical treatment of IBD in the elderly is a more controversial issue. In general, surgery is performed as an emergency procedure for acute life-threatening problems caused by IBD, such as perforation or severe bleeding. Other urgent reasons for operating include recurring or chronic complications such as obstruction, abscess, and fever. Failure to respond to a medical regimen may prompt elective surgery. These generalizations are also true for surgery in an elderly individual with IBD, keeping in mind two guiding principles. One is that surgery is not contraindicated by age alone. The second is that older people do as well as young people when surgery is performed electively rather than as an emergency. When an older IBD patient requires emergency surgery for an acute complication of IBD, surgery should not be delayed just because of the person's age.

Which operation is the best for the elderly person with IBD is beyond the scope of this discussion and, as in the younger subject, is best made by the surgeon based upon the individual needs of the patient.

PART 2

Supportive Treatments

15 // Nutritional Management

Nutritional deficiencies are common complications of IBD. This is not surprising considering the chronic nature of these illnesses, their tendency to begin in adolescence and young adulthood, and the fact that gastrointestinal symptoms are often made worse by eating. In addition, inadequate food intake, poor intestinal absorption, loss of nutrients across the damaged bowel, chronic diarrhea, and the potential for adverse drug-nutrient interactions all may cause nutritional depletion. Careful attention to diet and the use of modern techniques of nutritional support can prevent nutritional deficiencies and can actually help in the medical and surgical treatment of symptoms.

DIET AS A CAUSE OF IBD?

It is quite natural for individuals with IBD to look for a connection between the development of their bowel disease and the food they eat. Several studies have suggested the association between IBD and the consumption of certain foods, including refined sugar, cereals, fiber, milk products, protein, and others. However, research has not been able to confirm these associations, and at present no dietary factor can be implicated as a cause of IBD.

NUTRITIONAL DEFICIENCIES IN IBD

The most important reason for poor nutrition in IBD is inadequate food intake. Gastrointestinal symptoms such as nausea, abdominal pain, and diarrhea occurring at mealtimes can cause a decrease in appetite and food intake. Children and adolescents with IBD may not consume enough calories and other nutrients for proper growth and development (*See Chapter 12*). IBD patients may be placed on restricted diets that prevent adequate intake of specific vitamins and minerals if supplements are not used. For example, a diet low in dairy products, recommended because of lactose intolerance, may not provide adequate calcium. Low-residue diets restricted in fruits and vegetables may not provide adequate vitamins. Both types of diets may be deficient in calories.

Malabsorption of essential nutrients also may cause nutritional deficiency in people with Crohn's disease of the small intestine, especially in those who have had intestinal resections or extensive disease where bowel surface area may be inadequate for absorption. Resections or disease of the ileum have special nutritional consequences: bile salts, which are absorbed specifically in the ileum and which play an important role in absorption of dietary fat, may be lost in the stool, resulting in poor absorption of the fat soluble vitamins A, D, E, and K. Vitamin B12, also absorbed specifically in the ileum, may be lost because of ileal resection or disease, resulting in vitamin B12 deficiency if proper supplements are not used. Patients with small intestinal strictures or fistulas between loops of small bowel may develop an overgrowth of bacteria in the affected bowel loops, resulting in malabsorption of fat, vitamin B12, and other nutrients. Finally, some IBD medications may cause malabsorption of specific nutrients: corticosteroids interfere with calcium absorption, and sulfasalazine causes malabsorption of the vitamin folate. Cholestyramine, a bile acid-binding resin used to treat diarrhea in some patients with Crohn's disease, can interfere with absorption of the fat soluble vitamins.

IBD also results in excessive intestinal secretion of protein-rich fluids and loss of nutrients through the diseased gastrointestinal tract. Such a "weeping" of circulating proteins through the inflamed bowel wall, known as protein-losing enteropathy, contributes to protein depletion. Severe diarrhea causes depletion of electrolytes, minerals, and trace elements such as zinc. Gastrointestinal bleeding can cause iron deficiency anemia.

There is evidence that some people with IBD may need more of certain nutrients than normal individuals. Certainly patients with fever, infections, or those undergoing surgery have greater requirements for protein, calories, and other nutrients than patients who are less severely ill.

NUTRITIONAL THERAPY OF IBD

Your physician will attempt to manage your nutritional problems by maintaining an adequate nutrient intake while modifying your diet to decrease your gastrointestinal symptoms. The importance of correcting and preventing nutritional deficiencies cannot be overemphasized, since protein-calorie malnutrition and deficiencies of vitamins and minerals may affect the structure and function of the gastrointestinal tract. An IBD patient who is malnourished may enter a vicious cycle wherein the secondary effects of nutritional deficiency may worsen gastrointestinal symptoms and further compromise nutrient absorption. In addition, malnutrition will significantly retard healing of the inflamed and damaged bowel.

The composition and pattern of your diet must be modified to minimize stress on the diseased bowel. As with other digestive disorders, it may be helpful to eat frequent small meals to decrease the volume of food and gastrointestinal secretions that the damaged bowel must handle at any one time. Because protein-losing enteropathy is almost always present with active inflammation, your diet should include about 25% more protein than the recommended dietary allowance. You may need extra calories if you are severely ill or have significant malabsorption resulting in energy losses in your stool.

Many individuals will have subclinical deficiencies of vitamins, minerals, and trace elements that can be detected only by special laboratory tests. To remedy these deficiencies, many physicians recommend taking a multivitamin providing one to five times the recommended daily allowances of specific vitamins. Patients with malabsorption may need higher doses to prevent or correct micronutrient deficiency. Remember that all vitamin and mineral supplements are potentially toxic, and you should not take large doses of these unless they are prescribed and properly monitored by your physician. Individuals with Crohn's disease who have significant ileal disease or resection may require intramuscular vitamin B12 injections.

Modifications In Your Diet

A low fiber diet is often used in patients with narrowed segments of bowel to decrease the possibility of intestinal obstruction. Some physicians believe that a low fiber diet also helps to reduce the mechanical stimulation and irritation of the bowel while others have found that a high fiber diet may actually decrease symptoms in some patients with IBD. Dietary fiber, a term that refers to the parts of plants or vegetables that cannot be digested by the human gut, is composed of many different substances. Some of these substances, such as soluble fibers (guars and pectins) may decrease gastrointestinal motility and retain water. They can therefore be used to reduce the frequency of bowel movements in patients with diarrhea.

In the course of Crohn's disease, the active inflammatory process may cause an obstruction, particularly in the small intestine where the bowel lumen is narrower. Such active obstruction is usually associated with nausea, vomiting, abdominal pain, fever, and occasionally, diarrhea. Patients may be more comfortable with liquids while awaiting a response to medical treatment. When the obstruction is complete or almost complete, all oral feedings should be stopped until the obstruction is relieved. With improvement, the consistency of the diet may be increased progressively from clear fluids to full fluids, including blenderized foods, then to a soft diet, and finally to a regular diet. The purpose of these maneuvers is simply to prevent mechanical obstruction of a swollen, scarred, or narrowed channel by food particles. When the channel widens, or the obstruction is relieved, the consistency of the diet may be increased. In general, foods that are poorly digestible or high in indigestible fiber, such as corn, nuts, popcorn, or Chinese food, should be avoided if intestinal narrowing is present.

Malabsorption of lactose (milk sugar) occurs in many people with IBD, probably because the ethnic groups at risk for developing IBD are also those that tend to be lactose intolerant. Since dairy products are an important source of dietary cal-cium, protein, and calories, especially in growing children and adolescents, it is important that the possibility of lactose intolerance be investigated before re-stricting dairy products. Lactose intolerance is characterized by the occurrence of abdominal cramps, bloating, or diarrhea after ingestion of milk or milk products; a variety of tests for lactose intolerance is available in your hospital laboratory or physician's office. If you are lactose intolerant, you may treat your dairy products with a widely available bacterial lactase such as Lactaid® to make them tolerable.

Fat malabsorption contributes to diarrhea and, paradoxically, increases the risk for developing oxalate kidney stones. If you have significant fat malabsorption, your physician will probably restrict your intake of oxalate-rich foods (spinach, tea, rhubarb, etc.) and of dietary fats to about 70 gm/day. More severe restrictions are not helpful or necessary, and may even be harmful.

Nutritional Support

For some patients with severe IBD or extensive bowel resections, it may not be possible to meet nutritional goals with alterations of the normal diet alone. In this case, various types of formula diets and supplements can serve as the total dietary intake or as an addition to a restricted diet. Formula diets can be classified as:

1. *Meal replacement formulas* that are similar in composition to the normal diet
2. *Elemental or defined formula diets* that are generally low in fat and contain other nutrients in predigested or easily digested forms
3. *Modular supplements* that are not complete feedings, but are used to provide a specific nutrient to supplement a restricted diet or another formula

Individuals with moderate disease or limited intestinal resections usually prefer meal replacement formulas or modular feedings since they are generally more pal-atable and less costly than elemental diets. Elemental diets are reserved for pa-tients with severe malabsorption who cannot tolerate the fat contained in meal replacement formulas. Useful modular supplements include medium-chain tri-glyceride oil as a source of calories in patients with fat malabsorption, liquid or powdered protein supplements, and glucose polymers as a well-tolerated source of carbohydrate calories.

Enteral supplements can also be used to treat Crohn's disease. Recent studies suggest that elemental diets, often combined with antibiotics, may be as effective as steroids in reducing the symptoms of Crohn's disease. Some investigators be-lieve that the combination of an elemental diet and antibiotics decreases the im-mune stimulation of the gastrointestinal tract caused by normal fluid intake. How-ever, symptoms may reappear more quickly in patients treated with elemental diets than in those receiving steroids. Low-residue formulas are often used to treat patients with enterocutaneous fistulas high in the intestinal tract, since these diets are readily absorbed in the upper small intestine and will decrease the flow of intestinal contents. Formula supplements are especially useful in treating children with growth retardation caused by IBD. Reduced calorie intake is the main reason why these children fail to grow and develop normally, and use of the supplements often results in improved calorie intake and resumption of normal growth.

Since the unpleasant taste of some dietary supplements may make it difficult to consume enough calories, flavoring agents may be added. Formula feedings may cause diarrhea, gas, and cramps because they are so concentrated. Dilution of these products is usually successful in treating these symptoms, although larger volumes must obviously be taken. Some IBD patients learn to insert a nasogastric tube through which supplemental tube feedings can be taken and some take tube feedings at night while eating a restricted diet during the day.

Total Parenteral Nutrition

The ability to meet an individual's total nutritional requirements with intravenous feedings is known as total parenteral nutrition (TPN) and has been a major advance in the care of people with IBD within the last decade. TPN carries a greater risk of complications and is far more costly than enteral nutrition, and should be used only when formula diets and tube feedings have been unsuccessful or are not recommended. It is always preferable to use the intestinal route for nutrition whenever possible.

Several studies have suggested that TPN can be used to reverse immunologic and other abnormalities in IBD patients who are awaiting surgery, and may even reduce postoperative complications in some cases. Further research is needed to determine which patients will benefit most from preoperative TPN and to ascertain the appropriate length of nutritional therapy before surgery. Currently, preoperative TPN is generally recommended for about 7 to 10 days before surgery in malnourished individuals or in those who cannot eat for a prolonged period after surgery.

TPN and Bowel Rest as Therapy

TPN and bowel rest (taking nothing by mouth) may also play a role in the management of Crohn's disease unresponsive to medical treatment. Between 40% and 80% of patients treated in this manner will have a decrease in symptoms and be able to resume eating after 3 to 4 weeks of treatment with TPN and bowel rest. Long-term follow-up of those who respond initially to TPN is needed to determine the optimal duration of therapy. Even without this information, many physicians are now using home TPN to decrease the length and cost of a hospital stay.

The use of prolonged TPN and bowel rest is recommended only in patients with severe Crohn's disease unresponsive to medical treatment, and in those individuals who must avoid surgery because of previous resection or inoperable disease. TPN does not appear to be effective in the medical management of ulcerative colitis.

Only a few patients with ulcerative colitis treated with TPN and bowel rest avoid colectomy, and randomized controlled studies in ulcerative colitis have demonstrated no advantage of TPN over conventional medical treatment.

TPN can reverse the severe malnutrition associated with enterocutaneous fistulas in Crohn's disease, and often results in complete closure of the fistula. Closure tends to be temporary, however, and fistulas often reopen when oral feedings are resumed. Some IBD patients develop postoperative fistulas at the suture line after bowel surgery. These fistulas are much more likely to close permanently with TPN and bowel rest.

As previously noted, growth retardation in children with IBD is often the result of insufficient caloric intake. Some children with active bowel disease cannot eat enough to meet their nutritional requirements. This is particularly true when disease is active because the physician is avoiding high doses of steroids for fear of growth suppression. In these situations, TPN in the hospital or at home has allowed these children to consume enough calories to resume growing.

Finally, long-term home TPN is essential in individuals with Crohn's disease who have had extensive intestinal resection resulting in the so-called "short bowel syndrome." Home TPN can be used safely and effectively in many of these patients, permitting both nutritional and social rehabilitation. Long-term reliance on home TPN has identified a number of complications. These include newly recognized micronutrient deficiency syndromes, bone disease, liver and gall bladder diseases, and infections, as well as mechanical problems associated with long-term use of an intravenous catheter. For this reason, dietary modifications and enteral nutrition support are the first line of therapy before embarking upon the costly and somewhat risky approach of home TPN.

16 // Psychotherapy in IBD

All illness requires psychological and social adjustment. For patients with IBD, this may include coping with chronic or recurrent symptoms, working through concerns related to possible complications or surgery, or learning to deal better with life stresses that may aggravate symptoms. For most people, these adjustments are made with the support of family and friends, the clergy, physicians, and peer organizations such as the Crohn's & Colitis Foundation of America (CCFA; *See Chapter 17*). However, if the symptoms of IBD are incapacitating, or if these usual methods of support are inadequate, professional effort will be required to help make a satisfactory adjustment to the illness. Therefore, the use of therapists to help individuals deal more effectively with life stresses can play an important role in routine medical treatment. There are several situations for which psychotherapy may be helpful.

WHEN STRESSFUL EVENTS WORSEN SYMPTOMS

Although it is unlikely that stressful events and other psychosocial factors cause IBD, research and clinical experience indicate that these factors may lead to a flare-up of IBD, just as with other diseases. For example, animal studies show that changes in social environment can result in damage to internal organs, including the gastrointestinal tract. Interestingly, the first reported cases of ulcerative colitis in Bedouin Arabs occurred among a group who were relocated from their life in the desert to government housing. Perhaps the stresses of a more modern life style influenced the development of their symptoms. Research in a number of combined disciplines is providing evidence that social and psychological stressors modify the body's immune function and alter the release of various substances which, in turn, alter bodily function and the activity of disease.

Just how important stressors are in affecting your disease must be determined individually and in consultation with your physician. Many factors can play a role, and being under stress does not necessarily mean that your IBD will become more active. Furthermore, daily stresses often affect the function of the gastrointestinal tract and produce diarrhea or abdominal pain (the so-called "irritable bowel") without a change in the activity of the underlying IBD. If you or your doctor determines that your life stresses lead to discomforting or disabling symptoms, then professional help to reduce these stresses or your reaction to them may be beneficial.

WHEN STRESSES ADVERSELY AFFECT HOW YOU FUNCTION WITH YOUR ILLNESS

Life stresses and other psychosocial factors will affect *how* an illness is experienced. For example, in the face of some distressing event such as the loss of a job or an argument with a loved one, a person with IBD may feel a worsening of symptoms, and be less able to carry on daily activities. When the stressor is relieved, or the person is able to adapt to the stressor by mastering it, tolerating it, or minimizing its personal impact, the symptoms will improve, even without a change in disease activity. (Here, we make a distinction between *disease*: abnormalities in the structure and function of organs and tissues, and *illness*: the person's perception of ill health or bodily dysfunction.)

It is also important to consider the degree to which the disease or its treatment adversely affects your quality of life. In using the Sickness Impact Profile, a questionnaire that evaluates how people function with their disease, researchers have learned that those with IBD are affected primarily in their work, sleep and rest, recreation, social interaction, emotional behavior, and home situation more than in the areas of general mobility and body care. Family, friends, and health care workers who focus primarily on your medical symptoms may not fully recognize the total impact of the disease on your life. Whereas treatment of the disease through medication and surgery will improve these functions, your quality of life is also affected by attitudes such as the sense of control you feel in the face of illness, and types of coping strategies you can develop. These attitudes and coping strategies can be strengthened through proper education and by psychological treatment.

WHEN YOU OR YOUR PHYSICIAN RECOGNIZES A PSYCHOLOGICAL DISORDER REQUIRING TREATMENT

People with a serious medical illness like IBD can occasionally develop illness or anxiety disorders that require treatment (*See Chapter 11*). Whether these disorders result from or accompany IBD is usually impossible to determine. What is important is that they are recognized and treated appropriately. At times, even the person with IBD who has a psychologic disturbance may not be aware of its presence. If your physician recommends psychotherapy, try not to be defensive; it may be in your best interest to agree, since ultimately the treatment is likely to improve your overall health and ability to function. However, psychotherapy, if recommended, is not likely to be helpful unless you approach it willingly.

The type of psychotherapy depends on individual interests and needs.

Individual Insight-oriented Therapy

If you are a psychologically minded and motivated individual, insight-oriented, "one-on-one" psychotherapy is an appropriate option. This form of therapy offers the unique opportunity to learn about your perceptions and reactions to interpersonal relationships and life stresses in a supportive and nonjudgmental environment. Its goal is to help you develop the resources to modify attitudes and behaviors to future stresses and to find more adaptive ways to cope with the illness. The disadvantages are that not everyone is able or willing to make the necessary personal commitment, and the process can be expensive and time-consuming.

Short-term "Crisis" Therapy

If you generally feel and function well, but a specific crisis (such as a decision about major surgery or the loss of a close family member) leads to a difficult adjustment or to emotional difficulties, supportive counseling over a 4- to 6 week-period can be considered. The goal is to provide professional guidance and support until the crisis has resolved and you can return to normal functioning.

Family Therapy

In the face of chronic illness, family members must also adapt psychosocially; if this does not occur, family function may deteriorate. For example, if a spouse is called on to make personal sacrifices when the patient's health worsens, he or she may experience a sense of helplessness or anger. Expressing these socially unacceptable feelings is difficult, particularly if the spouse believes (usually unrealistically) that they will aggravate the patient's condition. Feelings of anger may smoulder or show up as withdrawal of support to the patient, or as anger directed toward the patient or doctor (for not being able to make the patient better). Similarly, as the parent of an adolescent child with IBD, you may harbor inappropriate feelings of responsibility for the disease and may then overcompensate for these feelings by being overprotective. In these situations, the therapist can help the family work to understand these feelings and ineffective interactions, and help the family strengthen its role as a source of mutual support.

Group Therapy, Mutual Help, Support Groups

This type of therapy is less expensive and is particularly useful when you are able or willing to discuss personal concerns in a supportive group environment. The group is organized and facilitated by a therapist who may select participants with similar difficulties or concerns, or by chapters of the CCFA and the United Ostomy Association (UOA; *See Chapter 17*).

Behavior Modification Therapy

Relaxation training, biofeedback, and self-hypnosis are techniques to help an individual achieve a greater sense of relaxation through reinforcement and conditioning. A therapist may also use behavior modification and cognitive psychotherapy to help a patient reduce maladaptive behaviors. The therapist first gets the patient to recognize these actions and helps to reinforce healthier forms of behavior. These techniques should be considered for the patient who would like to achieve "stress reduction" without addressing the possible underlying factors contributing to the tension state. You must be motivated to practice these techniques on a regular basis.

17 // Support Groups for the Person with IBD

In recent years, self-help or mutual support groups have gained rapidly in popularity. There are two fundamental concepts behind these groups: first, persons with a common concern can gain strength as a group by pooling their resources; second, persons with a problem in common can gain individual strength by communicating with others who have successfully overcome the same problem.

Crohn's disease and ulcerative colitis are the types of medical conditions for which these groups can be extremely beneficial. People with IBD often feel terribly isolated, as though there is no one who really understands what they are going through. Symptoms like chronic pain, weakness, diarrhea, and bleeding are not easily discussed, even among friends and family members. Few outsiders can appreciate the extreme anxiety associated with the need to be near a bathroom, which is experienced by many people with IBD. Participation in support groups may be the first time they have ever met and talked with another person with Crohn's disease or ulcerative colitis and shared their anxieties and problems in coping with IBD.

Many chapters of the CCFA have formed successful self-help or mutual support groups for patients, parents, singles or couples, and teenagers. Some support groups are led by volunteer lay members of the group, while others use psychologists or social workers as consultants. Support groups for people with IBD have been set up according to several different models. Two of the most common group models are described below.

The lay-led group is a small informal group or "rap" session led by a lay person who may share the same condition or experience with other members of the group. Since the leader is not a trained professional, and may occasionally suffer from "burn-out" or ill health, a co-leader is often advisable. Lay-led groups generally meet on a regular basis, weekly or twice a month, either in a meeting place or in someone's home. Frequent meetings help cement a feeling of trust and confidentiality.

Professionally-led groups ask the guidance of a mental health professional such as a psychologist or social worker as either group leader, group facilitator, or consultant. In these groups, the professional is usually selected because of his/her skill and experience in group dynamics and not because of expertise in a particular disease or condition. Group members understand far better than the professional what it is like to live with a chronic disease like IBD. For this reason, it is important for the core group itself to decide the extent of the professional's participation in the group. Some professionals could be used simply to get a group started and running, whereas others could be used to guide discussion in the group.

TOPICS FOR SUPPORT GROUP DISCUSSIONS

After the group is underway and members are beginning to get to know each other, new group leaders may worry that there might not be enough to talk about in group sessions, and that there may be long uncomfortable silences. Although experience with IBD support groups has shown that there is more than enough to talk about, some new leaders may feel more comfortable with a list of possible topics to introduce. The following topics have been used by support groups in some CCFA chapters; the questions can be used to help stimulate discussion.

1. *Reaction to Having a Chronic Illness.* What does it feel like to find out that you have a chronic illness? What was your first reaction? Did this change with time?

2. *Reaction of Friends and Family.* Who acts as your support system—parent, spouse, sibling, or friend? How did they react when you were first diagnosed? Did you get good advice from those close to you? Is it easy to ask for help when you need it? How does your support system react to long bouts of illness?

3. *Impact of IBD on Life Style.* Can you work, go to school, take a vacation, go out with friends? Have you missed work days or classes? How have the teachers or employers reacted to your illness? If you are single, how is your social life? Are there certain precautions you take if you know you will be taking a long car ride, not knowing where the next bathroom may be? Does you life sometimes depend on where the bathroom is?

4. *Dealing with Your Physician.* Is your doctor available when you need attention? Are all your questions answered? Have you been told about the possible side effects of your medications? Does your doctor spend enough time with you on the phone? In person?

5. *Feelings About Medical Treatment.* How do you feel about surgery, tests, having to take medications? How do you feel about trying new medications? Being part of a clinical trial?

6. *Feelings About Sex.* Do you have fears about something happening during sexual intercourse, fears of being unattractive, fears about having children? How open can you be with potential partners without scaring them away?

7. *Using the Illness.* Do you use your illness to get attention or pity? Is it a way to "cop out" when necessary? Do your reactions create problems in the family or with friends? When is psychotherapy a good idea?

8. *Sharing Coping Strategies.* Is it a good idea to carry an extra change of un-

derwear at all times, or a portable toilet in the car, or to check ahead to find where the bathrooms are located? Should a parent talk to teachers on behalf of a child to make sure of immediate access to toilet facilities, etc.?

Being able to speak about these concerns brings a tremendous sense of relief to the person with IBD. Some group members eventually become group leaders, and continue the support process by giving back to the new group members that sense of togetherness and support that they received and which is essential to coping with IBD. To assist you in starting or continuing a support group for IBD patients, CCFA publishes a manual, *Organizing a Self-Help Group for People with IBD*, which can be obtained by contacting the Foundation.

SUPPORT FOR THE PERSON WITH AN OSTOMY

Probably the single most important support service provided for IBD patients with ostomies is the Visiting Program sponsored by the UOA. After being certified as visitors, UOA chapter members are entered into a local pool of available visitors. Every time the chapter receives a referral for a visit, whether pre- or postoperative, or in the hospital or the patient's home, a Chapter Visiting Coordinator selects the most appropriate certified visitor from the pool on the basis of type of ostomy, age, sex, marital status, and life style. The referral is passed on to the matched visitor, who arranges the time for the visit with the patient and the nurse. During the visit, the person provides emotional support and gives nonmedical information and ostomy-related publications to the patient, while observing the rules and guidelines previously learned during visitor training. After the visit, the visitor will follow up with one or more telephone calls and sometimes another visit, if one is needed. The visitor will complete a report form to provide the chapter and ultimately the national organization with information about the visit, but at no time is the *confidentiality* of the patient compromised.

Before becoming a certified visitor, candidates must have had their surgery at least one year earlier, and must have the recommendation of their personal physician. They may then attend the chapter's next visitor training class. In addition to attending and participating in the class, a trainee will be interviewed by a person experienced in ostomy visiting. Upon successful completion of these requirements, the candidate is certified as an ostomy visitor.

Visitor training classes are conducted by most UOA chapters at least annually. UOA provides resource materials and a guide for the curriculum, as well as suggestions for instructors. Normally, as a minimum, a surgeon, physician, enterostomal therapy (ET) nurse, and an experienced visitor would participate in conducting a day-long seminar. Other professionals such as psychiatrists, pharmacists, and social workers may also participate. Each seminar typically presents information on ostomy anatomy, postsurgical care, skin care, ostomy appliances, and proper visiting procedures.

OSTOMY DISCUSSION GROUPS

Group discussions among persons with ostomies are another important support service provided by the UOA. At the monthly chapter meeting, sometimes as the main program but more often as a much appreciated addition to it, attendees assemble into discussion groups. In a normal-sized chapter, there probably would be separate groups for colostomates, ileostomates, and those having had alternate surgical procedures. Participation is purely voluntary, but most persons find that the groups provide an opportunity to exchange useful information and helpful hints on skin care, diet, equipment management, and appliances. Discussion often covers other problems involved with day to day living with an ostomy and interpersonal relationships. Whenever possible, a knowledgeable person, such as an ET nurse or long-experienced ostomate, is assigned to lead each discussion, both to provide the benefit of his/her knowledge and to ensure that the discussion does not lead into subjects that are more properly the domain of medical professionals.

For information on IBD and ostomy support groups, you may contact:

Crohn's & Colitis Foundation of America
444 Park Avenue South
New York, NY 10016-7374
(212) 685-3440, (800) 343-3637

United Ostomy Association
36 Executive Park, Suite 120
Irvine, CA 92714
(714) 660-8624

18 // Genetic Counseling: Is It Necessary?

Ulcerative colitis and Crohn's disease are not classic genetic diseases in which it is possible to predict who will develop them. There are no obvious inheritable metabolic abnormalities, chromosomal defects, or mutant genes. Moreover, there are no biochemical or genetic markers currently known for IBD. However, genetic and familial influences may play a role in 20% of patients with ulcerative colitis and 20% to 40% of patients with Crohn's disease. Usually, when IBD "runs" in the family, one additional family member (usually first degree relatives —parents, children, siblings) is affected; rarely, several may be involved. Such familial clustering of an illness does not necessarily prove the existence of a genetic mechanism, nor does its absence completely exclude this possibility. Infectious diseases may cluster, as can some noninfectious disorders because of similar life styles and cultural patterns within families. Indeed, the evolution of many diseases depends on the complex interaction of familial tendencies and external environmental factors. Each type of IBD tends to run true in affected families. Thus, ulcerative colitis in a family member is more likely when the initial patient ("proband") has ulcerative colitis, while Crohn's disease is more likely with a proband who has Crohn's disease. In 25% of affected families, both conditions are seen within the same family. IBD, especially Crohn's disease, also occurs among twins, even those living far apart. Classic genetic disease associations with IBD also are rare but they *do* occur; these include ankylosing spondylitis occurring with ulcerative colitis (*See Chapter 10*) and psoriasis with Crohn's disease.

Evidence supporting a genetic or familial association with IBD, therefore, is weak. For this reason, scientists currently classify IBD as a disease requiring the involvement of external, environmental, and noninheritable factors for its expression. The familial association may reflect a vulnerability to external or environmental factors, but not to the actual disease. This predisposition may vary from person to person and by ethnic group. In some surveys, the familial vulnerability to IBD appears increased among Jewish families. The external events that precipitate IBD are unknown and may include bacterial and viral infections, unknown and casual exposure to various foods or other toxins, antibiotics, and perhaps even severe stress. Current evidence favors an infection of the bowel.

What then is the practical significance of the familial association for the parent with IBD? Does it signify the need for genetic counseling? The answer to this question is no. There is no scientific justification for curtailing family size, for having an abortion, or for testing children in the absence of symptoms. There is no way to predict who will develop IBD and no medication to prevent its occurrence. Parents with IBD should support warm family relationships without fearing the possibility that their children might develop IBD.

Parents with IBD understandably will be more aware and more sensitive about digestive complaints among their children. In most cases, these digestive complaints are caused by the same things as in other children whose parents do not have IBD. An irritable bowel syndrome with abdominal pain, gas, bloating, diarrhea, or constipation is a common disorder in many American households. However, continuing symptoms of abdominal discomfort or cramps, diarrhea, fever, weight loss, or failure to grow are indications for a medical examination. Only rarely do these symptoms prove to be ulcerative colitis or Crohn's disease.

It is hoped that the investigations of the "familial IBD tendency" currently in progress will clarify the nature of this vulnerability and will facilitate either early protective intervention or complete prevention of the tendency to develop IBD.

PART 3

When Surgery Becomes Necessary

19 / Indications for Surgery in IBD

Both ulcerative colitis and Crohn's disease respond well to the available medications described in the first part of this book. Many patients have a benign course with only intermittent or occasional flare-ups and some have extended periods of inactivity (remissions). Unfortunately, in some patients with IBD, chronicity or complications may necessitate surgery. You should not consider surgical intervention something to be avoided at all costs, but rather as another way of treating your IBD. Even if your disease is mild or in remission, you should understand from the beginning what surgical options are available in case your symptoms should worsen in the future.

The purpose of this introduction is to provide you with a broad perspective of the reasons why surgery may be necessary in Crohn's disease and ulcerative colitis. Further details about specific operations can be found in Chapters 25 through 34.

ULCERATIVE COLITIS

Surgery may be indicated in ulcerative colitis as an elective procedure or in an emergency. In either case, the operation of choice is almost always colectomy (removal of the entire colon) since ulcerative colitis usually recurs in an unresected segment of colon. On the positive side, it is encouraging to remember that colectomy permanently cures ulcerative colitis. Inflammation does *not* recur in the small intestine, and there is no need for further medical treatment of IBD. However, since available medications usually control symptoms, most patients will not require a colectomy. However, since the possibility of colectomy always exists, it is important to understand what situations might call for this solution.

Emergency Indications For Surgery

If you have ulcerative colitis, you may be faced with the possibility that a colectomy and ileostomy are needed. Having to make such an important decision on short notice is very difficult. However, it is better to lose your colon than your life. After the life-threatening emergency has been eliminated with a colectomy, you should be restored to good health, and may then have the option of choosing one of the newer surgical alternatives (continent ileostomy, ileoanal anastomosis with or without reservoir) over the standard ileostomy that is usually performed during emergency surgery. The situations that might lead to an emergency colectomy include perforation, massive bleeding, fulminant colitis, and toxic megacolon.

Perforation

Perforation results when the ulcerations in the colon extend through its wall, causing a hole. Air and stool can then enter the abdominal cavity, producing peritonitis. If you have not been taking steroids, symptoms develop and progress quickly. However, if you are taking high doses of steroids, these signs and symptoms may be masked for a number of hours or days. In this situation, the diagnosis is made when a simple x-ray of the abdomen reveals "free air" in the abdominal cavity. When this is seen, you will be taken to the operating room as soon as possible and a colectomy will be performed. Perforation usually occurs in severely ill patients, and rarely occurs early in the course of disease.

Bleeding

Severe bleeding requiring emergency surgery is uncommon in ulcerative colitis and usually responds to high doses of intravenous steroids and to blood transfusions. Very rarely may bleeding be so sudden and massive that a colectomy has to be performed.

Fulminant Colitis

The most common situation prompting emergency surgery is fulminant colitis with severe diarrhea, bleeding, and fever. If this occurs, you will be admitted to the hospital, taken off all oral feedings, and treated with high doses of intravenous steroids, antibiotics, and perhaps TPN to supply your nutritional needs. Your doctors will watch closely for any complications. Although it may alarm you and your family, a surgeon is called in "early" in the course of fulminant colitis to help your physician decide on the proper timing for surgery if it is necessary. Many physicians, especially those in England, believe that if there is no improvement within 5 days, an emergency colectomy is indicated. Other physicians delay surgery for as long as 10 to 14 days to watch for signs of improvement.

Toxic Megacolon

In toxic megacolon, the colon loses its muscle tone, distends, and is in great danger of perforating. Most surgeons feel that toxic megacolon is an indication for emergency surgery. However, others feel that this complication can be treated medically with intravenous steroids, antibiotics, and colonic decompression using nasogastric, intestinal, or rectal tubes. If the colon returns promptly to its normal size, patients are often continued on medical therapy with the hope of a prolonged remission. However, after decompression, toxic megacolon may recur. Disease usually remains active and surgery is usually required.

When emergency surgery is performed in ulcerative colitis, it is common to remove the colon, leaving the rectum in place and constructing a standard ileostomy. After the emergency is over, the rectum can be used for one of the newer alternative procedures, or removed at a later date.

Elective Indications For Surgery

Intractability

An intractable condition is one that does not respond to medical treatment and therefore prompts surgery. People with intractable ulcerative colitis often have a poor quality of life and cannot participate in usual activities because of the need to be close to a bathroom and the fear of an accident. Many in this group also suffer from side effects of prolonged steroid use (*See Chapter 5*).

The person with ulcerative colitis who is unresponsive to medical treatment must be the one to decide when surgery is necessary. Many sufferers of ulcerative colitis will avoid surgery for long periods of time if they feel the symptoms and toxicity of medication are not affecting their lives significantly. Often, their ability to tolerate these adverse symptoms is caused by fear of colectomy and ileostomy. However some patients may not realize how sick they are and how their life styles have changed. Only after surgery, when the inflamed colon has been removed and their health returned to them, can they appreciate how truly sick they were. After surgery, it is not unusual for many people to say, "I should have done this earlier and not suffered so many years with my ulcerative colitis." Others will select surgery earlier in the course of disease because they see surgery as an end to the suffering caused by the disease. Therefore, the definition of intractability is different for each patient. It is important to talk with your gastroenterologist and a surgeon to understand what is entailed in the different kinds of surgery. The following chapters in this section will provide a guide for discussion with your physicians.

Risk of Cancer

The risk of cancer is a frequent indication for elective surgery. Individuals with ulcerative colitis involving the entire colon and those with disease for 10 years or longer have an increased risk of developing colon cancer. In this group of patients, periodic surveillance with colonoscopy is one way to discover cancers at an early stage or to look for dysplasia, which is cell changes that may lead to cancer. During colonoscopy, tiny tissue samples (biopsies) of the colon lining are removed through the colonoscope and sent to the pathology laboratory. An experienced pathologist can then determine if a cancer or dysplasia is present. If severe dysplasia is found and confirmed by an experienced pathologist, cancer is either present in another part of the colon or will develop in the near future. However, before colectomy is performed, a repeat colonoscopy and biopsy is warranted to demonstrate the persistence of dysplasia. Strictures of the colon in patients with ulcerative colitis are also potential indicators that cancer has developed.

CROHN'S DISEASE

Since Crohn's disease frequently recurs after operation, and since surgery never "cures" Crohn's disease, surgeons have become much more conservative about recommending an operation in patients who do not respond to medical therapy.

In order to work with your physician in determining the proper timing for surgical intervention, you should understand the "natural history" of Crohn's disease, its response rate to different medications, the likelihood of recurrence after operation, and the frequent success of surgery in returning you to a good quality of life. You should also understand that the type of surgery will vary depending on whether it is being done electively or to treat an emergency.

Emergency Indications For Surgery

The complications that usually prompt emergency surgery in Crohn's disease include bleeding, free perforation, abscess formation, fistulas (both internal and external), intestinal obstruction, and toxic megacolon. However, emergency surgery may be required in some patients even *before* a diagnosis of Crohn's disease is ever made. These patients, often in their teens or early 20s, develop the classic signs of appendicitis: fever, pain, and tenderness in the right lower abdomen. When the surgeon operates to remove the appendix, he/she finds Crohn's disease instead, usually in the terminal ileum. When this happens, the appendix is usually removed anyway, even if it is normal. In the hands of an experienced surgeon, appendectomy is safe and will remove the possibility of future appendicitis.

In rare cases where appendicitis is suspected, ileitis or colitis will be found which is not Crohn's disease. Certain bacteria such as Yersinia, Campylobacter, and Salmonella, as well as parasites such as the ameba, can mimic Crohn's disease. Cultures and smears of the bowel and its contents will usually provide the correct answer, and appropriate medical treatment will result in cure with no progression to chronic bowel disease.

Bleeding

Bleeding may occur from any segment of affected bowel in Crohn's disease but is most common with colonic disease. Regardless of whether the bleeding arises from the colon or small bowel, it typically presents as bright red or maroon-colored blood passed through the rectum. When such bleeding occurs, it usually does so in the first few years of illness and frequently responds favorably to hospitalization, transfusion, and steroids. If the hemorrhage does not stop, your doctors will order tests to try to localize its source, including endoscopy, nuclear medicine scans, and angiography (x-ray study of the blood vessels). If bleeding continues during angiography, the exact site of hemorrhage can usually be visualized and substances can be injected to constrict or block the bleeding vessel. Episodes of massive bleeding are frightening to patients and their families, but fortunately they are seen only in about 5% of patients. This kind of severe hemorrhage usually requires surgery.

Free Perforation

In this situation, a deep ulcer in the bowel wall produces a hole into the peritoneal cavity. Bowel contents from the small or large intestine will leak into this space, causing fever, severe abdominal pain, and tenderness; this syndrome is called peritonitis. X-rays of the abdomen usually show that the gas that normally is contained in the bowel has now passed into the peritoneal cavity. This "free air" is an indication for emergency surgery. If untreated, peritonitis causes rapid deterioration and shock. Fortunately, free perforation is a rare occurrence in Crohn's disease. The type of surgical procedure to be performed depends on the site of the perforation, how long it has been present before surgery, and the extent of the Crohn's disease (*See Chapter 33*).

Fistula and Abscess

Many patients with Crohn's disease require surgery because of fistulas and abscesses. Although the inflammatory process initially may be limited to the bowel wall, in many patients the inflammation will pass through the intestine and into the surrounding fat, producing a fistula or sinus tract. The sinus tract is a blind pouch, but the fistula, by definition, finds its way into another segment of bowel (enteroenteric fistula), into another organ such as the bladder (enterovesical fistula), or onto the abdominal wall (enterocutaneous fistula).

Sometimes there will be no place for the inflammatory cells to drain and infection builds up until an abscess is formed. An abscess is suspected by the presence of pain, fever, and localized tenderness. Its presence is confirmed by laboratory tests including an elevated white blood cell count (WBC) and a high erythrocyte sedimentation rate (ESR). An abscess may be diagnosed definitively with a sonogram and/or CT scan. Abscesses must be drained. If the abscess is in the abdominal cavity, surgery usually entails a major operative procedure with drainage of the abscess and resection of the diseased bowel. If it is not safe to remove the diseased bowel because the patient is very debilitated, then the abscess may be drained and a temporary ostomy created until the inflammatory process subsides. Bowel resection can be performed later when the patient's overall condition has improved. Abscesses can sometimes be drained percutaneously, by passing a thin needle through the skin and into the abscess cavity. The pus can be withdrawn by suction on the syringe. Often the needle is replaced by a drainage catheter for several days.

All fistulas are not equal and the presence of a fistula is not an absolute indication for surgery. The type of fistula is very important in decision-making. Entero-enteric fistulas may be tolerated by patients for many years without requiring treatment. Alternatively, symptoms may be intermittent and treatable by simple short courses of therapy. If the patient does not respond to medical treatment, a fistula may require surgical intervention. For example, an ileovesical fistula may cause periodic pain, burning on urination, and fever, symptoms of a urinary tract infection that should respond to treatment with antibiotics. If symptoms persist or recur frequently and no response is obtained with antibiotics, metronidazole, or 6-MP, surgery may be indicated. Therefore, in a fistula complicating Crohn's disease, the need for surgery must be individualized and will depend on the location of the fistula, severity of the symptoms, and their response to medical treatment.

Obstruction

Obstruction is usually a late manifestation of Crohn's disease. After years of inflammation, the bowel wall may thicken and eventually narrow so that food cannot pass through the involved segment. Signs of obstruction include noisy peristalsis, cramps, abdominal bloating, fullness, nausea, vomiting, and pain. You should learn to recognize the early signs of bowel obstruction, since without prompt medical treatment, surgery may be required.

One factor influencing obstruction is the type of food you have eaten. Obviously, if you eat a great deal of roughage and indigestible foods that do not easily pass through narrowed areas, obstruction may result. A soft diet without raw fruits and vegetables is recommended when obstruction is likely.

A second factor causing obstruction is inflammation. Although the bowel wall may be slightly narrowed because of chronic disease, superimposed acute inflammation tends to promote further obstruction. For this reason, your physician will usually treat any obstruction with medications, including sulfasalazine, antibiotics, or steroids. When the inflammatory process subsides, the obstruction may resolve and you can usually resume your normal eating habits.

The third factor in obstruction is intestinal scarring. Scarring may be caused by adhesions from prior surgery, peritonitis, or from the Crohn's disease itself. When the inflammatory process reaches the stage where the bowel is obstructed, then neither food restriction nor medications will be helpful. In such a case, surgical resection or dilation of the narrowed area is required (*See Chapters 30 through 32*). If treated early enough, intestinal obstruction may not require emergency surgery. In any case, you probably will be admitted to the hospital, given no food by mouth, and treated with intravenous medications until the obstruction resolves. In the hospital, a narrow, soft plastic tube probably will be passed into your stomach or intestine in order to decompress the bowel. If obstruction subsides, a decision regarding the need for surgery can be made. Obviously, if medical treatments are not successful in relieving the obstruction, surgery is indicated.

Toxic Megacolon

Toxic megacolon is a condition in which the colon becomes more severely inflamed, distends with gas, and eventually runs the risk of perforating. Although there is some evidence that medical treatment may help to alleviate this complication of IBD, most physicians feel that toxic megacolon is an indication for emergency surgery. Fortunately, toxic megacolon is not common in Crohn's disease.

Elective Surgery for Crohn's Disease

Intractability

Indications of intractability in Crohn's disease may include persistent symptoms such as fatigue, weight loss or pain, intolerable side effects of medications (especially steroids), and the need for significant dietary restriction. In reaching a decision to have surgery because of intractability, the patient consults with the physician about whether surgery can change the course of disease and when it should be performed. At certain stages of their lives, many people decide that it is time to have the diseased bowel resected so they can move on to the next stage, that is, going to college, starting a new career, or having children. After surgery, symptoms and the quality of life should improve significantly. However, the risk of recurrence is always present. In a given patient, it is not known whether Crohn's disease will recur within the first few years after surgery, many years later, or not at all (*See Chapter 35*).

Cancer Risk

The risk of cancer is not as high in Crohn's disease as it is in ulcerative colitis. Cancers and lymphomas, tumors arising in the blood-forming tissues, e.g., spleen and lymph nodes, have been found in patients with long-standing Crohn's disease. These intestinal malignancies can occur both in the affected and nonaffected areas of the small or large intestine. In the past, if a patient had Crohn's disease of the terminal ileum, the surgeon would attach the more proximal end of the small intestine to the transverse colon, thus bypassing the inflamed area and hopefully allowing it to heal. Perhaps the most famous person to have had this bypass operation was President Dwight Eisenhower. Although this method offered some symptomatic relief, it placed the patient at increased risk of developing cancer in the bypassed loop of bowel. Today, surgeons try to avoid this type of surgery and remove all the severely diseased bowel.

It may be difficult to find malignant areas in Crohn's disease, since they usually occur in segments of very inflamed and ulcerated bowel. Although colonoscopy may reveal some tumors in the colon, the incidence of colon cancer in Crohn's appears to be too low to warrant routine colonoscopic evaluation. Surgery is indicated in Crohn's disease patients with either cancer or lymphoma.

Growth Failure

Surgery is an option in children with Crohn's disease who have failed to grow while on medical therapy. Deciding whether to operate in this circumstance is a complicated decision that requires knowledge of the child's growth pattern before the onset of disease and potential for future growth. These can be evaluated by growth curve patterns and x-ray studies of the bones.

In recent years, pediatric gastroenterologists have shown that poor growth in children with Crohn's disease is largely the result of inadequate caloric intake and that adequate nutrition will allow these children to grow. Extra calories can be taken in through intravenous TPN, enteral feedings at night through a nasogastric tube, and liquid nutritional supplements. These nutritional therapies are sometimes effective in controlling the disease process as well as encouraging growth. The use of steroids in growth-retarded youngsters is a double-edged sword, since steroids can promote growth by reducing disease activity or interfere with growth by causing premature closure of the growth plates of the long bones.

Another factor in deciding if surgery is indicated for growth failure is the extent of the disease process. Obviously, if a small segment of bowel can be removed, thus allowing the child to grow, this approach might be considered early in the course of treatment. When there is extensive disease of the small or large intestine, however, surgery should be deferred and medical management should take precedence.

Although Crohn's disease is not curable, surgery is still a valuable form of treatment. Indications for surgery vary according to the site of disease, its complications, response to medications, and the patient's physical and emotional response to the disease. Both patient and physician must spend time discussing these factors whenever surgical intervention is considered.

REFERRAL TO A SURGEON

Most people with IBD who face an operation already know quite a bit about their illness and its possible treatments. However, even a knowledgeable person, when confronted with the need for an unexpected operation, may become confused and frightened. For this reason, it may be advisable for anyone confronted with the possibility of surgery to ask the gastroenterologist, "Who is the appropriate surgeon for me?", before asking the surgeon, "Which operation is for me?". In most instances, your gastroenterologist will be able to refer you to a surgeon who is at once communicative, concerned, and expert in the treatment of IBD.

Much understandable and useful information can be obtained from conversations with your surgeon before any planned surgery. These discussions can also help you to anticipate the degree of personal interaction, understanding, and compatibility you can expect from your surgeon during the perioperative period, the period immediately before, during, and after surgery (*See Chapter 20*). If you are not satisfied with the level of communication with the surgeon, or if your questions cannot be answered to your satisfaction, you may wish to consult another surgeon.

The surgeon can be even more helpful to you if he/she knows how much you can understand and accept about your disease, how anxious you are about the impending surgery, and what kind of support system you have among family and friends. With this information, the surgeon can help you to anticipate the effects your operation may have upon your feelings about body image, sexuality, and on family relationships and work status.

Anatomical Considerations

It is important for the surgeon to be aware of features of your particular anatomy that may influence the choice of surgery. These include abdominal scars, body shape, or physical disabilities such as limited eyesight, weakness, spasticity, or paralysis. For example, a surgeon may be reluctant to perform an ileostomy unless absolutely necessary in a patient with impaired vision, or may wish that cataract surgery be carried out before abdominal surgery. Conversely, the development of cataracts or osteoporosis resulting from high-dose steroids might necessitate an earlier decision for surgery in an attempt to bring the IBD under control and reduce or eliminate the need for steroid therapy. A woman with moderately active ulcerative colitis who wishes to have a child may elect to have a total colectomy before becoming pregnant, and thus avoid the risk of exacerbation of disease and possible loss of the pregnancy. The construction of an ileostomy may be affected by the presence of a deeply indented lower abdominal scar from a previous pelvic operation.

The Type and Stage of the Disease to be Treated

An accurate diagnosis and estimate of the extent of IBD is critical information in deciding which operation is to be performed. In all but a small percent of cases, it is possible to distinguish clearly between ulcerative colitis and Crohn's disease; the cases in question involve only the colon and a differential diagnosis cannot be made easily. Patients with ulcerative colitis should keep in mind that the entire colon is at risk for development of the disease. When surgery is required, the entire colon and rectum are usually removed because of the tendency for the remaining colon to become diseased. This type of surgery is the only available cure for the disease. Less extensive surgery (e.g., partial or subtotal colectomy) is performed only rarely when active ulcerative colitis is confined to the left colon (*See Chapter 29*).

In contrast, patients with Crohn's disease cannot be cured by surgery. Significant improvement can be achieved, often with operations to treat complications of the disease, and occasionally with larger resections of small or large intestine. Most surgeons are conservative in recommending an operation in Crohn's disease because of the tendency of the disease to recur and to require repeat operations.

20 / Talking to Your Surgeon

Preparation for surgery begins by meeting with your surgeon one or more times to discuss the type of operation you are to have, the expected benefits and risks, and the possible complications. You must ask questions that are important to you and be certain you are fully satisfied with the information. Some may feel insecure with this approach for fear of seeming ignorant or because they don't want to disagree with the doctor. However, it is your right to make an informed decision, since you will experience the results of that decision for the rest of your life.

Studies in support of this approach indicate that persons with IBD adapt best to their disease and to the results of surgery when they:

1. feel well informed
2. are given information that they believe is useful
3. feel comfortable talking with their doctor
4. are given enough time to have their questions answered.

This is because adequate knowledge and successful communication with the physician seem to impart a greater sense of control over what is to come. Although no one can truly determine disease outcome, studies indicate that it is the patient's beliefs rather than the actual circumstances that lead to a successful adaptation.

Listed below are some important questions to consider when meeting with your surgeon:

1. The reasons for the operation.
   "Why is the operation being done?"
   "Are there other options?" Patients should keep in mind that even surgical treatment may have several options. For example, there now are three very different types of ileostomies that can be constructed for ulcerative colitis patients who require a colectomy.
2. The technical aspects of the operation.
   "What is to be done?" Many patients find it helpful to view a diagram of the intestinal tract and the anticipated changes to result from the surgery.
   "Who else will be operating?" At a teaching hospital or large community hospital, it is usual for surgeons-in-training to be involved with the operation. In

all cases, your surgeon will be "in charge," but the degree to which he or she is actually operating or supervising will vary, and this can be negotiated.

3. The expected consequences.

"What will it feel like when I wake up?" A major source of anxiety in having an operation relates to postoperative pain; knowing what to expect will produce a better recovery. In one study, patients who were told where the pain would be felt, how intense it would be, and who were assured that pain-killing medication would be available if needed, required less postoperative sedation and went home sooner.

"How will my bowels function?" Removal of small or large intestine even without the creation of an ostomy will usually lead to looser and more frequent bowel movements. The degree of this expected physiological effect should be discussed before the operation. However, sometimes it cannot be determined until the time of surgery exactly how much intestine will be removed or whether a colostomy or ileostomy will be performed.

"What are the chances of a complication and which ones are most common?" Some patients may become frightened when hearing of the possible complications of a major operation. However, to obtain informed patient consent, it is required by law that surgeons discuss the most frequent complications (See Chapter 21). For elective operations, serious complications are infrequent, occurring less than 5% of the time.

"What limitations in activity will I have?" You can expect to experience a 4- to 6-week recovery period before returning to all usual activities. The long-term limitations vary with the type of procedure and your overall health status. In general, more than 90% of IBD patients who require surgery report better physical function, recreational capability, interpersonal (including sexual) relationships, and overall improved quality of life. This is because patients who require surgery usually have severe or complicated disease and poorer health status. Therefore, removal of the active disease or surgical treatment of its complications will improve quality of life. However, problems can occur. For example, if extensive surgery must be done in the pelvic area, impotence in the male or pain on intercourse in the female is possible.

4. The prognosis.

"Will this cure my disease?"

"What are the chances I might eventually need more surgery?" Remember that the surgeon can only base his/her prognosis on probabilities gathered from personal experience and the medical literature; you should never seek or expect guarantees. Nevertheless, if a decision is made for surgery, it is good to keep in mind that in most cases the benefits (such as freedom from risk of colon cancer, prevention of death from infection, relief of bowel obstruction, improvement in symptoms and quality of life) almost always outweigh the risks (perioperative death, postoperative infection, wound breakdown, inadequate clinical response).

5. Personal concerns.

Recently a group of investigators surveyed IBD patients to elicit their disease-related concerns, and of the top five concerns, four (having an ostomy bag, having surgery, worries about body image, loss of bowel control) were associated with surgery. It is natural that such issues are important to you, and they should be discussed before the operation, since your concerns may affect the final decision.

One important issue relates to the psychological consequences of having an external ostomy appliance. Whereas having an ostomy does not interfere with physical activity and is compatible with a normal social life, psychological adjustments need to be made. In one study, almost one-half of ostomates reported that sexual activity was less desirable because of the physical hindrance of the appliance, *yet more than 90% of the women and 70% of the men said that their spouses did not agree.*

For some patients, particularly adolescents and socially active young adults, adjusting to an ostomy may be difficult. For example, it has been shown that persons whose self-esteem is based largely on the function and appearance of their bodies are at higher risk for a poor postoperative adaptation to ileostomy. One patient, an adolescent with ulcerative colitis who was about to undergo colectomy, was fearful of being socially stigmatized by having an ostomy bag. The suitable option chosen for this patient was a colectomy with an ileoanal anastomosis (*See Chapter 27*). However, another ulcerative colitis patient, a middle-aged married truck driver, had greater concern about making frequent trips to the bathroom and having fecal soilage while on long trips. A colectomy with construction of a continent ileostomy (Kock pouch) was more desirable for him, since a small but substantial proportion of patients with the ileoanal anastomosis have diarrhea and soilage. For patients who have a difficult psychological adjustment to an ostomy, education and counseling by the physician or psychological referral can be helpful.

21// Giving Informed Consent

Your physician is required to obtain your informed consent before performing a procedure on you or instituting a new therapy for you. IBD patients are frequently asked to make informed consent decisions in several areas. Besides permitting a variety of surgical and endoscopic procedures, they must often decide whether to allow treatment with various drugs. Before embarking on any surgical, endoscopic, or drug treatment, you must ask questions. Reasoned decisions require information. Knowledgeable physicians want you to participate in your health care management and generally are eager to provide as much information as possible. In this way, the process of informed consent is satisfied.

WHAT IS INFORMED CONSENT?

Informed consent, as a legal doctrine, is relatively young; the first cases involving informed consent were reported in the late 1950s and 1960s. However, the ethical, moral, and humanistic values underlying informed consent are much older. Indeed, the right of a person to decide what should happen to him/her is a treasured personal right, and it is this right, the *right to self-determination*, that is the basis of the legal doctrine of informed consent.

The heart of informed consent is *disclosure*. In order for informed consent to be obtained, your physician must discuss certain elements of the proposed procedure or treatment with you. Over the last 30 years, two standards have developed that measure legally adequate disclosure. The first standard, still used in most of the United States, is the *professional or majority standard*, under which a physician must disclose to you those facts and elements that a reasonable physician would disclose under similar circumstances. This standard is set by the medical profession and must be established by an expert.

The second standard, used in a minority of the States, is the *lay or minority standard*, under which a physician must disclose to you those elements and facts that a reasonable person in your position would consider relevant in making an informed decision concerning a procedure or treatment. This standard is set by lay persons, not professionals, and is oriented more toward the needs of the consumer.

The essential *elements of disclosure* are basically the same under either standard, and include the following:

1. the nature of the proposed therapy or procedure
2. the potential benefits
3. the risks and potential complications with their relative incidence
4. the alternatives available, including doing nothing.

In obtaining your informed consent for a particular procedure or therapy, your physician will almost always request that you sign a permit or consent form. Do not mistake this form as your informed consent! Informed consent is not the same as consent. Informed consent is a *process* in which physician and patient interact in order to allow the patient to exercise his/her right to self-determination. Information is offered by the physician and appreciated by the patient. The patient's decision is based on knowledge and understanding of what has been explained about the proposed treatment.

Before signing any form, you must read it carefully. Be certain that the permit or consent form you sign sets out the procedure or therapy to which you have consented. Check to see that the risks and complications are listed accurately. If the form says that the risks and complications and alternatives of the procedure or therapy have been explained to you, be sure that they were. If, after reviewing the form, you believe that it accurately reflects the informed consent process in which you participated with your physician, it is reasonable to sign it as an indication that you have given your informed consent.

EXCEPTIONS TO THE NEED FOR INFORMED CONSENT

There are times when the legal requirement of obtaining informed consent is waived. These exceptions include the following:

1. emergency
2. waiver
3. incompetency
4. therapeutic privilege
5. legal requirement.

In order for the *emergency* exception to apply, there must be a life-threatening event in which there is too little time and opportunity to obtain informed consent. As with all of the exceptions, the emergency exception is interpreted narrowly. For example, a patient with peritonitis (infection caused by rupture of diseased bowel into the abdominal cavity) resulting from toxic megacolon needs emergency surgical treatment in order to survive. The surgeon must note the life-threatening situation at hand and must document the lack of opportunity to obtain informed consent because of time constraints. However, a sincere attempt should *always* be made to obtain informed consent for any procedure—if not from a severely ill patient, then from the patient's family or guardian.

A patient may *waive* the right to self-determination and instruct the physician not to disclose the nature of a proposed procedure, its risks, benefits, or alternatives. Such waiver is an exception to the physician's obligation to obtain informed consent, and in order for it to be valid, it must be made without coercion from anyone, and the patient must understand that he/she is relinquishing the right to know about the procedure or treatment.

The *incompetency* exception should be viewed with suspicion. Although a mentally incompetent person cannot give true informed consent to a procedure or treatment, the physician nonetheless has a duty to obtain informed consent from the patient's guardian before carrying out any procedure or treatment. In reality, incompetency is not an exception to the physician's legal duty to obtain informed consent.

The exception of *therapeutic privilege* is one in which the physician decides that the informed consent disclosure would be too harmful to the patient's decision. In this situation, the physician believes that the disclosure would cause the patient to make a decision to forego a necessary and worthwhile procedure or treatment. The physician then purposely fails to convey sufficient information to the patient to obtain legally adequate informed consent. For example, a physician might fail to tell a nervous male patient with long-standing ulcerative colitis about to undergo total colectomy that there is a small risk of impotence as a consequence of surgery. The physician justifies such incomplete disclosure by what he/she perceives as the patient's best interest, that is, the need for the colectomy. As you might guess, this exception is quite narrowly interpreted and, if used, should be accompanied by a thorough discussion with the patient's family, full documentation, and a psychological evaluation of the patient.

Finally, the exception of *legal requirement* or ruling is designed to balance the public welfare against the individual's right to self-determination. Imagine a mother of three young children who needs an amputation of her leg because of severe pyoderma gangrenosum (a form of treatment not usually required for this condition). She has refused surgery. Without the operation, she will likely die from sepsis. A judge might rule that she must have the amputation, despite her protestation. In so doing, he would balance her right to determine what should be done to herself against the public interest in her welfare and perhaps more important, the welfare of her young children. Such a ruling would eliminate the need for her informed consent before the procedure.

THE IMPACT OF INFORMED CONSENT ON IBD TREATMENT

In few other medical conditions is the physician-patient relationship as critical as it is in the treatment of IBD. It is important for both parties to have excellent lines of communication, mutual understanding, and empathy. IBD management can be as frustrating for the physician as it is for the patient, and the process of informed consent can be used to foster a better physician-patient relationship through communication.

CONSENT FOR SURGERY

In the process of obtaining your informed consent before any surgery, your physician must be sure to mention a variety of issues, including the fact that the surgery may not be curative, may need to be repeated, may disturb sexual function, and may result in certain physiologic irregularities of bowel function. It is far better that you understand the limitations of surgery beforehand than discover them afterward. Honest and forthright discussion should be the goal of the physician-patient interaction in making a surgical decision.

It is always a good idea to consider a second opinion for major elective surgery. For example, a woman with Crohn's disease and a vaginal fistula would benefit by obtaining several opinions before undergoing a surgical procedure. Should she have surgery at all? Will gynecologic surgery be necessary? What is the likelihood of cure? Is there a chance that she will develop recurrent fistulas? If so, what are the odds? Will she need a temporary ileostomy? How many procedures will be necessary?

These and many other questions in a case like this need careful consideration and require considered responses. This young woman might benefit from the expertise of several physicians from varied disciplines, including a gastroenterologist, a surgeon, and a gynecologist.

The informed consent process offers the physician an excellent opportunity to provide information and to show concern and empathy for the patient. Both physician and patient should welcome the opportunities for shared decision-making that the process of informed consent offers them.

22 // What to Expect Before, During, and After Surgery

With modern techniques of intravenous nutrition, potent methods of pain control, powerful broad-spectrum antibiotics, and a variety of new surgical techniques, a person need not be as fearful about entering the hospital for surgery. However, the advances in medical care and modern technology have made care in the hospital seem highly complex and understandably bewildering. Special skills and training are needed to provide such advanced technology. Skilled nursing personnel, nutritionists, intensive care teams, ostomy specialists, anesthesiologists, and medical and surgical specialists may all be involved in the care of one person hospitalized for surgery. Your attending physician is the person who coordinates the care you receive from these many skilled persons and who can help you to understand how each of these specialists can help you.

As medical therapy becomes more complex, patient education is essential to help you make informed decisions and to alleviate your anxiety before and during hospitalization. In addition to reading medical and lay literature, you should have frank discussions with your doctor to help you know what to expect during your hospital stay. This chapter can be used as a starting point for these discussions.

THE PREOPERATIVE PERIOD

With increasing pressure for cost containment, much of the preoperative care may take place before you even enter the hospital. Physical assessment, clinical testing, education, and some of the preparation for surgery may be done while you are an outpatient.

Physical Assessment

In preparation for surgery, a complete history is taken and physical examination is performed. Important active problems may require special evaluation before surgery. For example, a history of emphysema or heart disease may require consultation with a specialist to determine the importance of these problems and their impact on any planned surgery. Information about past operations, current medications, allergies, and any past problems with anesthesia is crucial. Any history of easy bleeding after a tooth extraction or small laceration also should be mentioned.

During the preoperative evaluation, certain consultations may be needed. An evaluation by a nutritionist is frequently obtained and special blood tests may be required to determine if you are malnourished. If necessary, a supplemental nutrition program can be started, ranging from the simple addition to the diet of high caloric liquid drinks to more complex dietary measures. In cases of severe malnutrition, intravenous feeding (TPN) can be used as the sole source of nutrition. This requires placing an intravenous catheter called a central line in one of the large veins of the body, usually located in the neck or chest (*See Chapter 15*).

If a colostomy or ileostomy is planned as part of the surgery, even if only temporary, an ostomy specialist will usually be consulted. This person, known as an ET nurse, will help in determining the best location for the ostomy (*See Chapter 23*). A properly chosen site should cause only minimal interference with work or social activities. The future ostomy site is commonly marked with an indelible ink that will not wash off during the preoperative cleansing of the abdomen.

After admission to the hospital, the nursing service will make its own assessment of any special nursing requirements you may have. In many hospitals, nursing floors are divided by specialties in an effort to concentrate the availability and need for specific nursing skills. As a result, the nurses on a general surgical floor are particularly accustomed to problems encountered during hospitalization for bowel surgery. Many of your questions can be answered by the nursing staff on your floor.

A preoperative assessment also will be performed by your anesthesiologist. After a review of your history, he/she will discuss the type of anesthesia that will be used, as well as its risk and complications. If you have any past history of adverse drug reactions, you should be certain to alert the anesthesiologist.

Clinical Testing

An array of laboratory tests are usually performed before surgery. A blood count, chemical profile, urinalysis, and blood clotting studies are generally routine. In addition, many people will need a chest x-ray and an electrocardiogram. Blood typing is always performed. Many patients worry about the risk of developing AIDS should a blood transfusion be necessary. Since 1985, all donated blood in the country is tested for the presence of antibodies to the human immunodeficiency virus (HIV). Therefore, the risk of developing AIDS from a transfusion is minimal. In some medical centers, patients have the option of banking their own blood or that of a friend or family member before surgery.

Other laboratory tests are performed as needed. For instance, pulmonary function tests might be done for someone with a history of asthma severe enough to require medication or hospitalization in the past.

Education

The preoperative period is also a time of intensive learning. It is natural to have many questions about surgery, anesthesia, and related matters, most of which can be answered by the hospital staff. Your gastroenterologist may always be consulted to discuss medical alternatives to surgery, evaluate specific problems, or assist in preoperative and postoperative care.

Preparations for Operation

Other activities that will occur during the initial hospitalization are the preoperative preparations, or "preps." If the planned operation is elective, you probably will be admitted the day before surgery. Timing of admission can vary, especially if the surgery is an emergency or if prolonged preoperative nutrition is needed. In such cases, a longer hospitalization may be needed to ensure that conditions for operating are optimal.

Intravenous fluids are commonly administered the evening before surgery. Fluids are administered through a catheter placed in a forearm or hand vein. The usual intravenous fluids contain dextrose (sugar), water, and electrolytes, such as sodium, potassium, and chloride.

To limit the amount of stool and bacteria in the bowel at the time of surgery, a bowel preparation including oral antibiotics will be started soon after admission. Two basic methods of cleansing the gut are used. The first is a series of enemas combined with oral laxatives. An alternate and increasingly popular bowel prep involves drinking a large volume of poorly absorbed liquid (such as Golytely® or Colyte®) that cleanses the bowel over a short period of time. Once the bowel preparation is completed, a clear liquid diet is usually prescribed until the midnight before the operation, after which nothing should be taken by mouth. The nursing staff will inform you if you may still take your oral medications.

Many people with IBD will have received corticosteroids for prolonged periods before surgery. When given for more than 2 to 3 weeks in a high enough dose, steroids can suppress the natural production of these hormones by the adrenal gland. As a result, the adrenal gland cannot provide the increased levels of steroids required during a stressful time, such as an operation. If needed, steroids may be given as an intravenous or intramuscular injection before, during, and for several days after surgery. On the night before operation, most surgeons will prescribe an optional sleeping pill. Of course, pain medications are given as needed.

To decrease the risk of developing a postoperative pneumonia, respiratory therapy is often started before surgery. Training is frequently given with the incentive spirometer, a device that encourages the patient to blow air forcibly from one tube into another, increasing lung capacity. If you are a cigarette smoker, be sure to discontinue smoking at least 5 to 7 days before surgery. This will help greatly in preventing postoperative respiratory infections.

The day of surgery may involve some waiting. Surgical schedules are usually made up the prior afternoon or evening. However, since emergencies are common, the actual schedule is often modified. Once you are called to the operating area, a preoperative intramuscular injection of a narcotic and sedative is usually given. Sometimes, atropine is used to reduce secretions in the mouth and nasal passages. Intravenous antibiotics are administered as needed. Only after all this activity are you finally ready for surgery!

THE INTRAOPERATIVE PERIOD

Anesthesia

Once you are in the operating suite, the anesthesiologist will begin preparations for inducing anesthesia. Anesthesia is usually accomplished in two steps. Intravenous sodium pentothal is commonly used to initiate anesthesia while other intravenous and inhaled medicines will be used to maintain sleep during the operation. During surgery, muscle paralysis is maintained with a medication such as succinylcholine. After a satisfactory level of anesthesia has been reached, other catheters and intravenous lines can be placed without causing you pain. A small plastic tube, called an endotracheal airway, is inserted through the mouth and into the trachea. This tube is used to ventilate the lungs by means of an attached mechanical respirator during the operation. Oxygen and anesthetic gases are pumped in and out of the lungs to mimic normal breathing. While you are asleep, blood will be sampled from the arterial circulation to determine that sufficient oxygen is being given.

The type of anesthesia may be modified to meet your individual needs. For example, if general anesthesia poses an unacceptable risk, as in cases of severe emphysema, and if the planned surgical procedure is minor, your surgeon and anesthesiologist may elect an alternative to general anesthesia, such as spinal or epidural nerve blocks. These are accomplished by injecting a locally active anesthetic into the area around the lower spinal canal. Complete absence of feeling below the level of the injection can be obtained with these methods.

Monitoring and Catheters (Tubes)

In addition to keeping you free from pain, the anesthesiologist monitors your blood volume and cardiac status. In high-risk situations, and sometimes during a long and complicated procedure, special tubes are inserted in central veins and arteries to measure various cardiovascular functions and may remain in place for several days after surgery. Blood pressure and blood volume are closely monitored. Large amounts of intravenous fluids may be administered, but a blood transfusion will be administered only when there has been significant blood loss or anemia.

Measurement of urine volume is another important way to determine fluid requirements and is accomplished by placing a soft rubber tube (Foley catheter) into the bladder through the penis or the urethral opening just above the vagina. Usually this catheter is inserted in the operating room after induction of anesthesia. The end of the catheter has a small balloon that is inflated with water to prevent it from slipping out. Urine drains through the tube by gravity into a plastic bag. It is customary to have a urinary catheter in place for several days after surgery. This eliminates the frequent need to get out of bed to urinate and helps minimize discomfort.

Whenever surgery involves removal or manipulation of bowel, as it does in IBD, a nasogastric tube will be used. This soft plastic tube is narrower than the width of a pencil and is passed through the nose and into the stomach before or during the operation. Suction applied through the tube keeps the stomach decompressed during surgery, removes fluid secreted by the stomach, and minimizes postoperative bowel distension. The nasogastric tube often irritates the back of the throat, but this discomfort passes a few days after removal of the tube. This tube is usually removed once normal bowel function has returned and you begin to pass gas. The endotracheal tube, mentioned earlier, can also cause a mild sore throat for a few days. Sucking on lozenges or ice chips is soothing and helps reduce the irritation. However, it may be 1 or more days before these are allowed.

Preps, Sutures, Drains, and Catheters

After induction of anesthesia, the surgical team begins by shaving the abdominal and pubic hair as required and then scrubbing these areas with an antiseptic solution. After opening the abdomen, your surgeon will proceed with the planned operation. A wide variety of synthetic suture materials can be used to rejoin cut tissues and close the abdominal wound. Some of these materials are slowly absorbed by the body, while others remain intact. Increasingly popular are new stapling devices that use metal clips to hold the tissues together (Fig. 1). Many surgeons prefer to close the edges of an abdominal incision using a stapling device because closure is rapid and incisions heal quite well. High tensile-strength wire is used in areas subject to tension and physical stretching, such as internal tissues of the abdominal wall.

Drainage catheters are placed around the areas of removed bowel. Seepage of fluids commonly occurs in these areas and can cause a wound infection if not adequately drained. These drainage tubes are commonly inserted into the abdominal wall at a site separate from the primary surgical incision and usually result in another very small scar. Drains and sutures are removed during the postoperative recovery period with only minimal discomfort. A slight burning while urinating is not uncommon after removal of a Foley catheter, and this may persist for a day or so. Burning for longer than a few days may be a sign of a urinary tract infection and should be mentioned to your doctor.

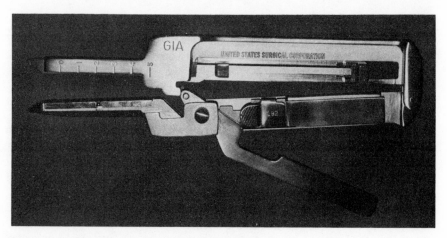

FIG. 1. Stapling device used to close surgical incisions.

Recovery Area

When the operation is finished, the anesthesiologist will gradually reduce the level of anesthesia, allowing slow return of normal function. Once you are breathing effectively without assistance, the endotracheal tube can be removed. Pain medications and light sedation are maintained to avoid discomfort. You will then be moved to the recovery area for careful observation. This is a specialized intensive care facility designed for short-term care. A highly trained staff of doctors and nurses will monitor all vital body functions while checking for any complications such as bleeding or respiratory distress. When your condition is stable, you will return to the nursing floor to begin your period of postoperative recovery.

THE POSTOPERATIVE PERIOD

The time needed to recover from surgery will depend on the severity of your illness, the extent of your operation, and other factors such as your nutritional status, age, and co-existing medical problems. Most people recover from surgery in a gradual fashion within 2 weeks. The usual course is a continued reduction in pain, the gradual return of bowel function, and a daily increase in activity. Of course, any complication can prolong hospitalization.

Intestinal Function, Diet, and Nutrition

Entering the abdominal cavity to examine the intestines causes a temporary paralysis of the bowel, called postoperative ileus. When part of the large or small bowel is removed, the resultant ileus can be of longer duration and may last at

TABLE 1. *Home-going instructions for abdominal operations*

1. Soft bland diet for the first month, unless instructed otherwise
2. Further diet instructions will be given at your postoperative visit
3. Try eating six small meals a day
4. Alcoholic beverages only in moderation
5. Climbing stairs allowed
6. May drive in 10 to 14 days, but do not go alone the first time. Avoid driving while on pain medications
7. Daily baths or showers okay and recommended
8. Dressings: Apply small soft gauze dressing over incision, and change as needed at least daily

   Other: _____

9. Any activity that causes pain should be avoided
10. Avoid lifting weights greater than 30 lbs
11. Avoid physical exercise that puts a strain on the abdominal muscles, e.g. sit-ups, press-ups, jogging, for 3–4 months
12. Bowel instructions:

    a. Avoid any foods that cause you diarrhea or gas

    b. If you are given antidiarrheal medication in the hospital, dosage may need to be adjusted if you experience diarrhea or constipation

    c. It is normal to have more gas or gas cramps after discharge from hospital. Avoid those foods that cause you to have gas

    d. It is normal to have some good days with respect to diarrhea and some not so good days. It takes your body time to adjust after surgery

13. *Acceptable foods*

Acceptable foods	*Foods to avoid*
Lean meats	Spicy foods
Chicken	Greasy foods
Fish	Onions
Turkey	Raw vegetables
Soups	Raw fruits
Mashed potatoes	Carbonated drinks
Bread and butter	

least several days. During this period when there is no peristalsis, fluids taken by mouth or secreted by the stomach cannot pass down the digestive tract and need to be removed by a nasogastric tube. Suction is applied to this tube through a wall-mounted or bedside vacuum device which can be disconnected for a brief interval when you are able to make trips to the bathroom or take short walks. Although eating or drinking will not be allowed, some surgeons will permit small amounts of ice chips or hard candies to soothe an irritated throat. Intravenous nutrition is often continued until the return of normal digestive function.

Your doctors will be listening to your abdomen for bowel sounds, an indication that intestinal function is returning. Passing gas and an improved appetite are other signs of recovery. Once intestinal function has returned, the nasogastric tube can be removed, and you can begin to eat again. Your diet will be advanced slowly over several days, starting with sips of water and progressing to clear liquids such as apple juice and broth, full liquids like puddings and ice cream, and ultimately to soft solid meals.

Pain Control

Careful control of pain is a fundamental part of helping you through the postoperative period. With modern techniques, pain relief can be easily accomplished. However, you should not wait for pain to become unbearable before asking for medication. Although you should not hesitate to ask for sufficient medication to ease your pain, you should not take medications frequently enough to become dependent on them (*See Chapter 3*).

Activity

You should try to get out of bed and even walk as soon as possible after your operation. This helps to reduce the risk of postoperative pneumonia and quickens the return of intestinal function. Before going home, the staples or sutures used to close the abdominal incision will be removed and replaced with small adhesive strips. If your surgery involved an ostomy, training sessions and ostomy supplies will be provided by the ET nurse. Before discharge, you will be given home care instructions (Table 1).

23 // What to Expect After Ostomy Surgery: The Role of the Enterostomal Therapy Nurse

The ET nurse is an integral part of the team providing care to the person who has had ostomy surgery. ET nursing was created as a specialty within the health care profession during the last 2 decades. The ET nurse provides direct patient care to persons with ostomies, teaches patients how to care for their stomas, and is a strong patient advocate. After successful completion of an accredited Enterostomal Therapy Nursing Education Program, the ET nurse is prepared to provide the highest level of this specialized nursing care.

HOW THE ET NURSE CAN HELP

Whether temporary or permanent, an ostomy alters body function, necessitating physical and psychosocial adaptation. Through skilled teaching, communication, and empathy, the ET nurse guides you and your family through the process of rehabilitation.

It is preferable that you meet with the ET nurse *before* surgery, when your greatest need is for information about the operation and its consequences. The ET nurse begins by making a thorough assessment of all your needs. The plan of care begins with educating you and your family, expanding on the information previously provided by the other members of the health team. The ET nurse provides information about the disease process, the intended surgical procedure, the resultant ostomy, and its effects on your life, including diet, clothing, activity, and personal relationships. The ET nurse uses a variety of techniques such as individual patient and family sessions, printed material, demonstrations, teaching models, play therapy for children, and a variety of audiovisual material (Fig. 1).

In the preoperative period, the ET nurse also begins to identify your particular emotional needs, evaluates your response to other life stresses, and develops plans to identify and assist those who may require additional support to adjust to the ostomy. Often just being available to answer difficult questions is of greatest benefit.

The ET nurse will carefully assess your abdomen and select the most appropriate site for your stoma. Based on your body build, location of scars, certain ana-

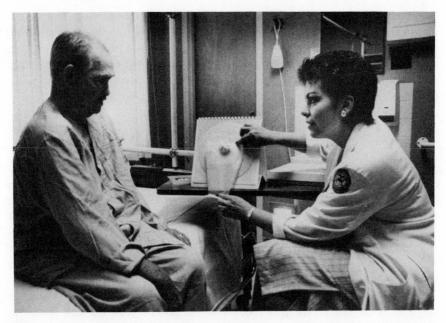

FIG. 1. An ET nurse begins the education process with a patient about to undergo ostomy surgery.

tomic landmarks, and how you wear your clothing, the ET nurse will select and mark the area where the stoma will be placed.

THE OSTOMY IMMEDIATELY AFTER SURGERY

Postoperatively, you will be wearing a skin barrier (a wafer that adheres closely to skin around the stoma) and a clear, drainable pouch to collect bowel contents which is attached to the wafer with a seal. The skin barrier protects the skin, and in some cases provides additional wearing time for the pouch. The pouch is clear so the stoma can be inspected daily and has an opening on the bottom that allows drainage and measurement of its contents. Many types of pouches and skin care products are available to meet your individual needs.

Immediately after surgery, the color of your stoma will range from pink to deep red. It may appear quite swollen but usually shrinks soon after surgery. The skin barrier and appliance should fit snugly around the stoma so that the skin is not exposed to the intestinal contents, which will cause irritation. Maintenance of skin integrity is an essential aspect of stoma care, and the ET nurse will spend quite a bit of time teaching you the proper skin care techniques.

The pouch and barrier stay on for 3 to 5 days after surgery, during which time the ET nurse will teach you how to empty it. Afterward, he/she will teach you how to change the appliance. Your greatest challenge will be learning how to care for your ostomy. Understandably, you may feel awkward, disgusted, or unwilling at first. These normal feelings resolve with time, patience, and practice. Written instructions will make this process easier. It is very helpful to be visited by a person with an ostomy who can talk to you as someone who's "been there." Such ostomate visits can be arranged through the UOA (*See Chapter 17*).

GOING HOME WITH YOUR OSTOMY

It is normal that you feel anxious about your new ostomy and your ability to empty and change the appliance on your own after leaving the hospital. Before discharge, the ET nurse will answer practical questions about bathing, how to wear particular articles of clothing, what to eat and what not to eat, odor control, and adjustment to the home situation, returning to work or school environments, and even about intimate sexual relationships. Family members should be included in teaching sessions whenever possible to help them become familiar with the ostomy and to provide additional emotional support.

If you are not able to care for yourself and your ostomy, the ET nurse will arrange for home health care as needed. You will also be provided with written instructions, supplies, resources for obtaining additional equipment, a phone number, or a clinic appointment for follow-up visits. Many ET nurses now practice independently or in home health care agencies and are easily available.

For further information on ET nursing, please contact:

International Association for Enterostomal Therapy
2081 Business Center Drive
Suite 290
Irvine, California 92715
(714) 476-0268

24// Psychological Preparation for Surgery

Surgery is a stressful event, both physically and psychologically. However, psychological preparation before surgery can be helpful. Several clinical studies have shown that education and behavorial forms of preparation lead to: 1) reduction in anxiety before and after surgery, 2) reduction in the amount of anesthetic agent required, 3) reduction in postoperative pain medication requirements, and 4) shortening of the hospital stay.

There are several methods of psychological preparation that you can use to prepare for surgery or any other medical procedure:

1. Obtain adequate information about the procedure and its effects, including the expected postoperative sensations. This can be accomplished through a discussion with your surgeon (*See Chapter 20*), and by reviewing patient educational materials (booklets, videotapes, etc.). By knowing what to expect, you will develop a sense of control over future events. However, for some patients, being "overbriefed," or receiving too much information may raise anxiety. It is important to let your surgeon know when you are satisfied with the amount of information you have received.

2. Use cognitive techniques. These coping methods involve using techniques of distraction, calming self-talk, or reinterpretation of the significance of events (cognitive reappraisal). For example, by learning to focus on the benefits of the surgery, the distressing concerns are "blunted" and are perceived as less frightening.

3. Use behavioral techniques. Behavioral methods include relaxation training (e.g., muscle relaxation exercises) to reduce anxiety or increase pain tolerance and self-care behaviors (e.g., deep breathing techniques) to acquire some control over the rehabilitation process and facilitate physical recovery. One example is progressive muscle relaxation:

1. Take three deep breaths, exhaling completely with a verbalized sigh.
2. Breathe slowly and rhythmically.
3. Concentrate all attention on relaxing successive sets of muscles. Begin with the tips of your toes and slowly move up to your legs, pelvis, abdomen, chest, arms, and finally to the muscles in your forehead. Feel the release of tensions as the muscles go limp.

4. Think of pleasant, relaxing thoughts: a peaceful mountain scene or the rhythmic motion of the waves on the beach.
5. Finish with 3 deep breaths.

   4. Involve the family. Family members should be involved in your preparation for surgery, not only to help you get through it, but to ease their feelings of helplessness. In one study, patients with Crohn's disease reported that working through and sharing the difficult experiences brought the family closer together. Family members can stay with you before and after the surgery, take care of your needs, and monitor your comfort during the recovery period.

PRACTICAL MATTERS

There are many practical issues and problems that may arise before you enter the hospital to have surgery. Hopefully, these matters can be settled in a thoughtful manner, well before hospitalization. This section will outline some major areas of concern and will provide guidelines to help you make plans before surgery.

Informing Your Employer

Most employers are sympathetic when an issue concerning an employee's health arises. If you are about to have surgery, your employer is entitled to know how long you will be in the hospital, the length of time you will be convalescing at home, and when you expect to return to work, either part-time or full-time. Your surgeon can give you an estimation of just how long recuperation will take. Many employers are more understanding about an employee's illness if they are kept informed and involved about the pending hospitalization.

Before you enter the hospital, it is always a good idea to plan ways in which your responsibilities can be covered during your absence. You should be prepared to present to your employer alternative strategies for reassigning or redistributing work to help minimize the impact of time lost while you are recovering. You may be able to remain normally productive until just before surgery. Just as you must think positively about the likelihood of the operation restoring you to health, your employer can reasonably expect that your job performance may actually improve as soon as your health is restored. You need to be sure that he/she does not expect too much too soon. It may take as long as 4 to 6 weeks to recover fully from abdominal surgery.

School

If you are a student, you should inform your teachers as early as possible about your surgery and the length of time you may be out of school. Teachers are usually very supportive and will help you plan ways in which you can keep up with your assignments. Before surgery, it may be possible to arrange for classmates and teachers to provide notes and assignments that you can complete while you are recovering. It is often possible to arrange for make-up examinations and formal tutoring if you are out of school for a long time.

Household Responsibilities

If you are the person in your family who is responsible for maintenance of the home and/or for child care, try to arrange well in advance of surgery for babysitters and housekeepers if you need them. This is also the time for parents and in-laws to lend a helping hand. Don't be afraid to ask for help; family and friends often need to hear from you about the specific ways they can be helpful.

Handling Your Personal Business

You should try to put your personal affairs in reasonable order before you enter the hospital. Check your health insurance policies to be sure of which services are covered and which are not. You may need to advise your health insurance carrier about plans for hospitalization and surgery, since some policies require a second surgical opinion with documentation from your physician before hospitalization. Without this information, reimbursement of hospital costs may not be approved. Remember to have the necessary medical insurance identification cards and/or your policy numbers with you when you enter the hospital.

Before any planned surgery, you should check in with those individuals who play an important role in your personal affairs, such as your accountant, personal lawyer, professional partners, colleagues, and close friends. At times, key responsibilities such as the payment of bills must be delegated to another family member to ensure that rent or mortgage payments and other important bills are paid on time. It is also reasonable for the head of a household to be sure that other family members (usually a spouse) know where important papers and documents are stored.

Physical and Emotional Preparation

You should try to be as physically and emotionally ready for surgery as possible. This is a good time to stop smoking, maximize caloric intake, and to exercise to maintain or improve muscle tone. Any of these steps will help you to recover more rapidly after the operation. To help boost your morale after surgery, encourage family and close friends to visit, but don't be afraid to set appropriate limits about hospital visiting. A member of your family might help you set guidelines so that friends do not "drop in" unexpectedly. You will not feel much like entertaining visitors soon after surgery, since you will be uncomfortable and drowsy from sedation.

Finally, it is important that you feel positive about yourself before and after surgery. It might be a good idea to get a haircut or even a new hairdo before being admitted. Women might bring cosmetics and plan to use them soon after surgery. Hospital barbers are often available to shampoo and cut hair. Keeping up your appearance will help you to feel better about yourself and may help you to recover more quickly.

PREPARING YOUR CHILD FOR SURGERY

Because of their more limited knowledge and incomplete emotional development, children and early adolescents are particularly vulnerable to adverse psychological effects from the surgical experience. As a parent you help determine what the young person needs to know and how much support is needed, depending on his/her level of intellectual and emotional development.

Since most operations performed on children with IBD are elective, there is usually adequate time to prepare the young patient for surgery. Preschool children should be told about the need for hospitalization shortly before admission, whereas older children can be notified in time to allow them time to think out questions they may want to ask. Every child should know the name of his/her doctor and be able to see the doctor daily in the hospital.

Obviously, for those patients who require emergency surgery, only limited preparation is possible. In this situation, it is even more important that the medical personnel act in a caring manner to comfort the parents and the child. The normal tendency for a child to have nightmares, loss of appetite, hyperactivity, or difficulty in falling asleep after returning home can be offset to some extent by reducing the stress and unpleasantness of hospitalization. Once again, a cooperative and friendly staff is essential.

How the Surgeon Can Help

A discussion of the planned operation with both the parents and the child is extremely important. Since even the thought of surgery on a child is anxiety-producing for parents, after explaining the procedure the surgeon may ask you to describe in your own words what will be done and why. This will help him/her to determine if you have understood the explanation. Your child should be permitted to ask questions since this helps to clarify any misconceptions and allay fears. Anatomical drawings or models are helpful, and the area of the surgical incision can be indicated on a doll as well as on your child's belly. Your child must be reassured that only the diseased parts of intestine will be removed and that no external or visible parts of his/her body will be cut off.

Since young children tend to fantasize that an operation is punishment for bad behavior, the surgeon should stress that surgery is necessary to treat the illness, and that the overwhelming majority of young people who require surgery for IBD show marked improvement and soon return to school and normal activities.

Hospitalization and surgery cause marked anxiety in the preschool child because of separation from parents and friends, loss of control in a new environment, and fear of injury and death. This can lead to depression, refusal to eat or speak, and the expression of regressive behavior, such as loss of bowel and bladder control, thumbsucking, clinging, and temper tantrums. Fear may be alleviated by a preadmission trip to the hospital where procedures for admission, nursing care, anesthesia, operating room, and recovery room can be seen and even rehearsed in play therapy with a team consisting of a nurse, play therapist, and social worker. In some hospitals there is even a puppet with a constructed stoma! Objects that children will come in contact with during their hospitalization can be brought into play therapy situation. These include a stethoscope, blood pressure cuff, operating room caps, masks, gloves, bed pan, oxygen and anesthesia masks, intravenous tubing, nasogastric tube, urinary catheter, and thermometer. The use of toy doctor and nurse kits and dolls allows hospital-based play and gives the child a feeling of some control over his/her new environment.

Hospitalization

When children are admitted to the hospital before surgery, they should be allowed to bring toys from home and wear their own pajamas. Visits by family members are to be encouraged. Often arrangements can be made to place a day bed in your child's hospital room so that you can spend nights with your child. Parents should be allowed to accompany the child to the x-ray department as well as to the operating room to allay fears of abandonment.

Any procedure that involves pain or discomfort must be described honestly and realistically before going into the treatment room (e.g., intravenous tubes, passage of intestinal tubes, removal of sutures). Your child will also be more cooperative when an intravenous line is inserted if he/she has seen other children who have similar ones in place. The use of central venous lines provides a pain-free method of supplying calories, vitamins, and electrolytes for young patients who cannot achieve adequate nutrition orally. These catheters can stay in place from days to months with a low complication rate. The fact that the child does not have to be "stuck" daily for intravenous therapy is a great advantage.

Children should not be told that they will be "put to sleep" before the operation because of its special meaning regarding pets who are "put to sleep" by veterinarians. Instead, they can be told that they will take a "special nap." Children must be reassured that they will not wake up until the operation is over and that they will wake up in the recovery room, usually wearing an oxygen mask.

PART 4

Operations for Ulcerative Colitis

25 / Proctocolectomy and Ileostomy

Surgery is the only available treatment that can bring about a complete cure and permanent relief from the symptoms of ulcerative colitis. However, most people with ulcerative colitis and their families live in fear of this curative procedure. Some of this anxiety is realistic, since perhaps 15% to 20% of people with ulcerative colitis will require surgical treatment and surgery does cause pain, some risk, and "lost" time for recuperation. More importantly, surgery for ulcerative colitis entails significant changes in bodily function and the physical and psychological adjustments that accompany these changes. On the other hand, many of the fears about surgery and the quality of life after surgery are often based on sketchy knowledge or outright misinformation.

Since fear of the unknown is usually worse than reality, the following explanation of surgical procedures and their results is presented to allay your anxiety. For those who are doing well with medical therapy, in whom operation is only a possibility for the future, peace of mind is the goal. For those in whom surgical treatment is an imminent consideration, detailed knowledge is essential to help you choose or reject a surgical approach to your disease, and to help you make an intelligent, informed choice among the different surgical procedures.

INDICATIONS FOR OPERATION

First, you must understand why surgery is necessary. The indications for elective or urgent operation have been discussed in detail in a previous chapter. To summarize, they are failure of medical treatment to relieve symptoms, the presence of intolerable side effects of medications, or the development of life-threatening complications. Although this sounds simple and straightforward, deciding that medical treatment has truly failed requires much careful thought and exhaustive discussion among the patient, the doctors, and, frequently, the patient's loved ones.

The following case history recounts one individual's experience with ulcerative colitis and describes how he decided to have an operation. His story illustrates the concept of failure of medical treatment in a lucid and vivid personal way.

121

My ulcerative colitis began rather innocently when, at the age of 34, I noted some blood on my undershorts after jogging. I was referred to a surgeon who performed a sigmoidoscopy and diagnosed an anal fissure. He prescribed suppositories, the use of which relieved the symptoms in less than a week.

There was no further trouble until about a year later when I noted some blood in the toilet water and on the tissue after a bowel movement. The same surgeon noted a limited and mild proctitis and referred me to a gastroenterologist for further treatment. With the use of sulfasalazine and a brief course of steroid enemas, all symptoms disappeared.

At this point in my life I was happily married and we had three sons aged 6 years, 3 years, and 6 months. Aside from being a bit overweight, I had been in excellent health and active in athletics. I was succeeding in business, involved in community affairs, and enjoying my family life to the fullest. Although I had some appreciation that I had a condition that might recur from time to time, I did not worry too much since I was informed that flare-ups were treatable and their number could be reduced by the continued use of sulfasalazine.

During the next 3½ years, I had periodic recurrences of rectal bleeding which were treated with steroid enemas, admittedly somewhat less effectively each time. Clearly, the disease was progressing subtly. However, I probably was not fully aware of this on a conscious level, perhaps from a desire not to confront the fact that I had a chronic disease. My colitis had not caused me any pain, interruption of my work, or disruption of my family life.

In the summer of my fifth year with ulcerative colitis, at the age of 39, I became quite sick with my first and the only major acute flare-up of my condition. I ran a fever, became extremely weak and, most distressing, I had multiple large liquid, bloody stools each day, sometimes with loss of complete control. A barium enema indicated that the disease had moved further up the colon. During this siege of illness I was unable to work for close to 3 weeks, lost 15 pounds, and experienced a substantial reduction in my energy level. I was begun for the first time on prednisone. Although I began to feel better, it became clear to me that things were different and, in one form or the other, my symptoms were here to stay. The biggest change was that my bowel movements still were quite frequent, averaging 5 to 10 per day. Furthermore, I was not able to sleep through the night since I needed to get up 2 to 3 times for bowel movements. My rather profound fatigue also persisted and, among other things, it interfered considerably with our love life. Nevertheless, I never considered or thought of surgery at this point since the symptoms, although unpleasant, were tolerable.

By the next summer I began to have severe abdominal cramps in the evening. X-rays done at this point showed what was presumed to be pseudopolyposis; this was confirmed by colonoscopy and biopsy, which revealed no precancerous signs. My doctor raised the issue of surgery at this point. I was very much against the idea and obtained a second opinion from a well-known gastroenterologist. He strongly recommended operation, pointing out that the operation would cure the disease and relieve all discomfort. Intellectually, I understood his reasoning, but emotionally I was not prepared for what I considered a radical change in my life, with a possible change in my physical self-image. In consultation with my doctor and two uncles who are internists, we decided to try to continue medical treatment for another year and take stock at that point. I felt that I could tolerate the symptoms for this period of time. Furthermore, I was told that cancer was not an immediate danger and it appeared that the dose and duration of treatment with steroids were not sufficient to make me particularly vulnerable to their side effects. I vowed to take extra good care of myself, to get plenty of rest and to shed some of my excess weight. Also, in conjunction with my physician, I hoped to be able to reduce the prednisone dose, preferably getting on to an alternate day schedule.

The year was difficult. I had severe abdominal pain almost every evening and occasionally during the day. Although I continued to play tennis and golf, I could not jog for any appreciable distance. I slowly began to accept the reality that the alternative to operation was living the rest of my life with pain and a low energy level, the need to be near a bathroom at all times and the possibility in the future of developing cancer of the colon. Although the thought of operation was still very alien and gave rise to many mental images that made me feel uncomfortable, I began to explore the option of surgery more seriously.

It was important to me that I be in control of this decision-making process. I would need access to good information and people resources. In addition to my own gastroenterologist and my two uncles, I spoke with another G.I. specialist and two expert surgeons who described the various surgical procedures. Eventually, I met with or spoke by telephone to several patients, some of whom had undergone conventional ileostomies and others some of the alternative operations. Obviously, my wife and I spoke at length about these matters. Although the fantasies with which I had been preoccupied still made me feel somewhat self-conscious and uncomfortable, it slowly became apparent to me that only by having an operation could I live my life satisfactorily.

WHICH IS THE "BEST" OPERATION?

As the end of this patient's narrative suggests, the consideration of operation is more complex today than in previous years because there is a choice of available procedures. No single operation is "best" for every patient. Which operation you should have depends on the extent of your disease and the quality of life you want. In subsequent chapters, each of the various operations currently in use for ulcerative colitis will be described and the results, advantages, and disadvantages of each will be discussed. Matters relating to preparation for any of the operations are considered in greater detail in Chapter 22.

TOTAL PROCTOCOLECTOMY AND ILEOSTOMY

Total proctocolectomy, by its nature, requires the construction of a permanent ileostomy. In this section we will describe the conventional procedure that is completed with a standard (Brooke) ileostomy. Total proctocolectomy can also be performed in conjunction with a continent ileostomy (Kock pouch), which is described in a subsequent chapter. Proctocolectomy with standard ileostomy is discussed first because it was developed first, has a long "track record," and is the "gold standard" with which the alternative operations are usually compared.

The Ileostomy

The ileostomy is the most important external change after a proctocolectomy (Fig. 1). For this reason, a great deal of attention is paid to choosing its proper placement on the abdomen. As shown in Figure 2, the ileostomy is usually placed

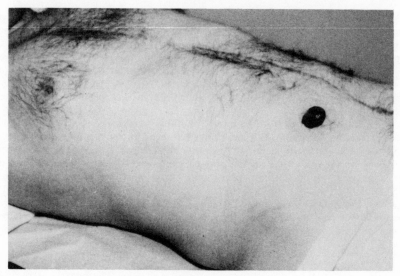

FIG. 1. Typical well-placed ileostomy (with the appliance removed) several weeks after operation.

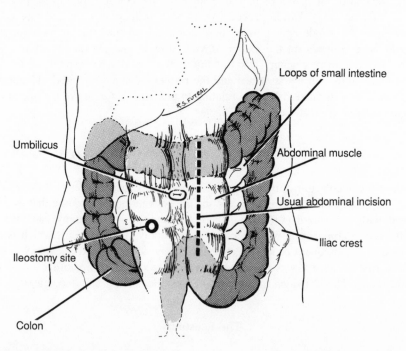

FIG. 2. Abdominal wall with the underlying intestinal organs. The usual site in the right lower abdomen for construction of a conventional ileostomy is shown, as is the usual placement for the abdominal incision.

in the right lower quadrant of the abdomen because this is where the ileum is located. The exact location on the skin is chosen so that the faceplate of the appliance does not interfere with the "belly button," the bony prominence of the pelvis, scars, and natural creases. This location also makes the appliance inconspicuous under clothing and prevents the faceplate from becoming detached when the thigh is flexed. The chosen site is then outlined with an indelible marker on the skin.

How the Operation is Performed

The performance of a total proctocolectomy consists of three main steps: 1) removal of the abdominal portion of the colon through an abdominal incision, 2) construction of the ileostomy, and 3) removal of the rectum. This involves a separate incision in the anal area. Sometimes the rectum is left in place (subtotal colectomy or total abdominal colectomy) with the intent of removing it during a subsequent operation or using it at a later time for one of the alternative operations.

There are two ways of positioning the patient on the operating table, depending primarily on the surgeon's preference. In the first or sequential method, the abdominal portion of the colon is separated from the rectum and removed, temporarily leaving the rectum in place. The ileostomy is made and the abdomen is closed. The patient is then repositioned to complete the operation by removing the rectum. In the second or synchronous method, the patient is placed on the operating table so that the abdominal and rectal portions of the operation can be completed without repositioning the patient.

Barring special considerations, the abdominal incision is usually made on the patient's left side to leave room for the construction of the ileostomy and the subsequent application of an appliance (see Fig. 2). The colon must be freed from its attachments to the surrounding structures all the way around from the right to the left side before it can be removed by cutting and tying off its blood supply. When the colon has been freed and its blood supply has been tied off, it is removed by cutting the ileum and placing an intestinal clamp across it. In Figure 3, the abdominal portion of the colon has been removed, leaving the entire small intestine and rectum. Clamps have been placed across the cut ends of the ileum and rectum before construction of the ileostomy and completion of the operation, either by removing the rectum or finishing it as a subtotal colectomy.

Completion as a Subtotal Colectomy

As mentioned before, subtotal colectomy may have been planned preoperatively because of the nutritional or medical condition of the patient, or his/her preference not to have the rectum removed. The decision to perform a subtotal colectomy can also be made during the operation, either because of the condition of the bowel at operation or a change in the patient's general status.

If subtotal colectomy is chosen, the colon is freed and removed as shown in

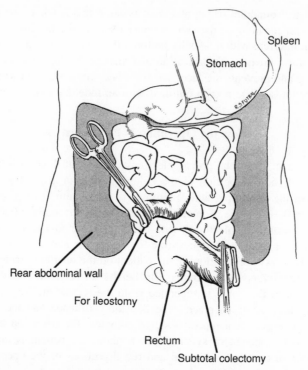

FIG. 3. The abdominal portion of the colon has been removed. Clamps have temporarily been placed on the last part of the ileum before construction of the ileostomy and on the rectum before its removal or completion of the operation as a subtotal colectomy.

Figure 3. There are two ways of dealing with the cut end of the rectum. The first method is to close it with sutures and replace it into the abdomen (Fig. 4). The second is to bring the cut end of the rectum to the abdominal wall, making it a nonfunctioning colostomy, or "mucous fistula." Obviously, a mucous fistula is not a true fistula in the sense of a disease complication. There is no unanimity of opinion as to which of these two methods is better. Closing the end of the rectum and leaving it in the abdomen prevents the annoyance of a draining mucous fistula. On the other hand, making a mucous fistula avoids the risk that the diseased end closure might break down.

After the colon is removed, all that remains to be done in a subtotal colectomy is to construct the ileostomy and to close the abdomen. Construction of the ileostomy will be described and illustrated below.

Completion as a Total Proctocolectomy

If the whole colon and rectum are to be removed in one operation, the rectum is removed after the abdominal portion of the surgery is completed. The rectum is

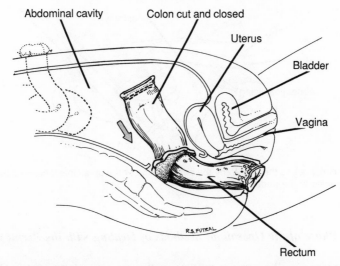

FIG. 4. In a subtotal colectomy, the severed end of the rectum has been closed with sutures and replaced in the abdomen, to be removed at a later date. This diagram of a female patient shows the relationship of the pelvic organs to the remaining rectal stump.

freed from its attachments to the bones of the pelvis and the urogenital structures, i.e., the uterus and vagina in the female and the bladder and prostate in the male. In contrast to the proctocolectomy performed for cancer, this dissection can be performed very close to the rectal wall, which helps preserve the nerves governing sexual function. If the operation is being done by the sequential method, at this point the surgeon will remove the abdominal portion of the colon. The cut rectum will then be placed in the pelvis (see Fig. 4) and removed during the perineal phase of the operation after the abdomen has been closed and the ileostomy has been constructed. If the operation is done by the synchronous method, the rectum is freed and the entire colon and rectum are removed without transection.

Construction of the Ileostomy

The ileostomy is fashioned by making a round opening in the skin and then in the abdominal wall, through which the end of the ileum is passed (Fig. 5). A portion of the ileum is made to protrude from the skin surface and then the end of the bowel is turned back on itself like a cuff and sewn in place (Fig. 6). As a result, a small protuberant stoma is created (see Fig. 1) so that the intestinal contents drain into the appliance without seeping under the faceplate. This method was described many years ago by an English surgeon, Professor Bryan Brooke, hence the name Brooke ileostomy. This simple technical innovation, together with the development of modern ileostomy appliances, makes recovery from surgery and postoperative rehabilitation much more rapid and trouble-free than it was years ago.

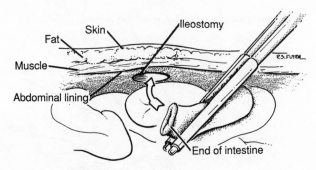

FIG. 5. In constructing the ileostomy the severed end of the small intestine is passed through a round opening in the abdominal wall.

Perineal Phase of the Operation: Methods of Dealing with the Perineal Wound

The surgeon usually removes the rectum through an incision in the skin around the anus. In the case of the sequential operation, after the abdominal incision is closed, the rectum is dissected until the portion detached in the abdominal phase of the operation is reached; the rectum is thus entirely free of its attachments and can be removed. In the case of the synchronous procedure, these two steps can be performed together while the abdominal incision is still open, and the rectal removal is completed after that of the colon. The removal of the rectum leaves a comparatively large, open space, the perineal wound, which then must heal.

The perineal wound may be packed with a dressing to help stop any bleeding, left open or partially closed with drains to promote drainage of accumulated serum and blood. The perineal wound heals by "secondary intention," i.e., by contraction of the tissue and ingrowth of the skin. This process is analogous to the healing of any laceration or incision that has not been stitched; the process takes several weeks to several months and requires frequent sitz baths, irrigations, and

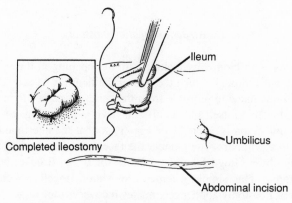

FIG. 6. The stoma is fashioned from the protruding end of the ileum.

dressings. A newer method that reduces healing time is to close the wound completely with sutures and to use temporary suction catheters to remove any blood or serum. Immediate suturing may prevent poor healing, the so-called persistent perineal sinus.

Postoperative Recovery

Because of the manipulation of the intestine in this or any abdominal operation, the bowel is more or less temporarily "paralyzed" and does not function normally, a phenomenon termed postoperative ileus (*See Chapter 22*). Because of this ileus, the ileostomy usually does not function for several days. Eating is not allowed during the period of ileus since it would cause abdominal distension, pain, nausea, and vomiting. Therefore, the body's need for fluids, salts, and other nutrients is met by intravenous feeding. Many surgeons use a nasogastric tube to remove gas and secretions, thus minimizing abdominal distension. As intestinal activity returns and the ileostomy starts to function, the nasogastric tube is removed, and eating can be resumed, starting with liquids and then progressing to a regular diet when appropriate.

Usually a urinary catheter is used to keep the bladder collapsed and out of the way during the operation. The catheter also serves to monitor the adequacy of fluid intake and output postoperatively and allows recovery of the bladder muscle which itself may have a period of postoperative "paralysis." The catheter is removed within several days to a week. Many surgeons administer intravenous antibiotics on the day of operation but discontinue them soon after unless required to treat an infection. If steroids have been given, they are tapered as quickly as possible. The high-dose steroids, together with the fact that the body is rid of the badly diseased colon, often make the patient feel amazingly well almost immediately. Occasionally, however, as the steroid dose is tapered there is sometimes a bit of let-down, but this is very transient.

The main thing that distinguishes recovery after a colectomy from many other operations is the need to learn how to care for the ileostomy. When you feel well enough to move about freely in bed, the nurse and ET nurse begin to familiarize you with your ileostomy, its function, the appliances, and other equipment needed for its care. You will first observe how the pouch is emptied, how the ileostomy is cleaned, and how appliances are changed, after which you will be encouraged to perform these tasks yourself. Discharge from the hospital (usually in 1 to 2 weeks) typically coincides with your ability to demonstrate independence in the care of your ileostomy (*See Chapter 23*).

AFTER RECOVERY: WHAT CAN BE EXPECTED?

A number of studies have shown that after removal of the diseased colon, a person with ulcerative colitis has the same life expectancy as any other person of the same age and sex. Tangible proof of this statement is the fact that a growing number of insurance companies are now willing to underwrite unrated life insurance and, in some instances, even issue disability coverage. The current mortality risk of total proctocolectomy is low, about 1% or less, and approaches that of a gall bladder or ulcer surgery.

If colectomy and ileostomy have such positive results, why is it so difficult for some patients to accept? Obviously the "price" is the fact that a person must learn to live with and accept the ileostomy—which is clearly a trade-off. This sounds much worse than it really is. The trade-off is an ileostomy instead of pain, constant diarrhea, fatigue, steroid side effects, and planning life's activities around the location of bathrooms. Also, sexual function is preserved in the vast majority of patients with colectomy and ileostomy.

Exactly what is life like with an ileostomy? The best way to understand the quality of life after ileostomy is to speak with people who have had the procedure. It is fair to say that most patients are amazed and comforted by what they see and hear. The fact that normal childbirth is possible and that well-known athletes have ileostomies only serve to dramatize the fact that ileostomies are not physically limiting. Ileostomates are auto mechanics, businessmen and women, factory workers, salespersons, executives, lawyers, and doctors.

Would one of the alternatives to total proctocolectomy and ileostomy be a better choice? For some people the answer is "yes," depending on individual goals and, in some instances, on the severity of disease. People clearly differ in their priorities. If the goal is the fastest, most certain restoration to health and "getting on with my life," a proctocolectomy and ileostomy are usually the answer. If a major objective is body image and the avoidance of an external appliance, one of the ileostomy alternatives should be considered. In general, the alternative operations are longer, more complicated procedures. More than one operation may be required and there is more "down-time" for achieving the ultimate result. After recovery, there is usually more need to watch your diet, a greater chance you will need medication, and a higher rate of future complications. Finally, if an ileoanal anastomosis or continent ileostomy is not satisfactory, subsequent conversion to a standard ileostomy is not straightforward. This is because at least a foot of ileum will have been sacrificed in the creation of the pouch and cannot be reused. As a result of this shortened bowel, the ileostomy discharge would be more liquid than usual.

An option for the undecided patient in many instances can be the subtotal colectomy and ileostomy, which leaves the rectum in place, so that the ileostomy can be experienced firsthand without "burning all the bridges"; the rectum will still be available for any of the alternative operations. Revision to a continent ileostomy (Kock pouch) is always possible whether or not the rectum has been removed.

Many people regard proctocolectomy and ileostomy as the "gold standard" operation for ulcerative colitis since it has been extremely effective in restoring health and has stood the test of time. However, there are obvious drawbacks to an ileostomy, and surgeons have since developed several satisfactory alternatives. Each of these alternative operations will be discussed in detail to help you decide whether they are right for you.

26 / Ileorectal Anastomosis

Many people with ulcerative colitis are discouraged from having definitive surgery, namely, proctocolectomy, because of their natural concerns about having an ileostomy. Historically, the first alternative to an ileostomy was ileorectal anastomosis. This operation consists of removal of the colon to the point where the colon joins the rectum. The small intestine remains intact and its lower end, the terminal ileum, is then connected to the upper end of the rectum. The last 6″ of the large intestine (rectum) are thus preserved, enabling defecation by the normal route (Fig. 1).

Ileorectal anastomosis was popularized by the British surgeon Dr. Stanley Aylett and is sometimes called the Aylett procedure. He observed that the inflamed rectal mucosa improved significantly in most patients after this operation; however, criticism of this operation was considerable in the 1960s for several reasons: an inflamed, diseased rectum was left in place, the remaining rectum was at risk to develop cancer, and further surgery to remove the rectum was practically inevitable. With accumulated experience, we now know that some of these concerns can be minimized by proper patient selection and improved surgical technique.

PATIENT SELECTION

There are several factors to consider before ileorectal anastomosis can be recommended in the surgical treatment of ulcerative colitis. These include age of the patient, appearance of the rectum, the condition of the anal sphincter muscles, and preexisting perineal disease or cancer.

Age

Some authorities have advised against the use of this operation in children because of the risk that cancer may develop in the retained rectum over so many years. Nevertheless, if the operation is performed in a young person, periodic proctoscopic surveillance with biopsy provides a measure of safety. Reduced

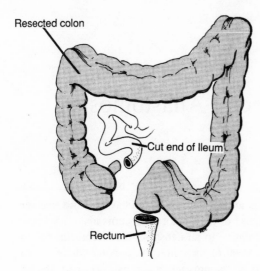

Resected colon

Cut end of Ileum

Rectum

FIG. 1. In ileorectal anastomosis, after colectomy the terminal ileum is connected directly to the cut end of the rectum, enabling defecation by the normal route.

sphincter muscle tone in some elderly patients makes it wise to examine this function to help select the best candidates for this operation.

Appearance of the Rectum

About 10% of patients with ulcerative colitis have a rectum that is relatively clear of disease. Patients with a relatively healthy and distensible rectum are good candidates for an ileorectal anastomosis. The degree to which the rectum can be expanded or stretched is judged in two ways: evaluating how much the rectal wall balloons out when air is instilled during proctoscopy, or by measuring how much air the rectum can hold before the patient experiences a strong urge to expel it. The greater this volume, the better the results. In other words, the more narrowed, rigid, and diseased the rectum is, the less likely that the operation will be successful.

The State of the Sphincter Muscles

Because varying amounts of diarrhea can be anticipated after ileorectal anastomosis, it is important to know if the anal sphincter muscles work normally. A history of sphincter injury (such as perineal laceration during childbirth) or poor anal function makes a good result less likely.

Perineal Disease or Cancer

Perineal disease is unusual in patients with ulcerative colitis. If present, however, especially if there is an active perianal or rectovaginal fistula, ileorectal anastomosis should not be performed. If dysplasia or cancer is present anywhere in the colon, but especially in the rectum, ileorectal anastomosis is *not* recommended. It is mandatory that this operation be followed by periodic proctoscopic examination to monitor the possible development of cancer in the retained rectum.

PERFORMING THE OPERATION

In about 75% of cases, the operation is done in one session and temporary ileostomy is not required. However, a temporary ileostomy may be needed if the colitis is very severe, if the patient is very ill, malnourished, or has complicating medical illnesses, if the operation has been unusually difficult, or if the healing capacity of the anastomosis is questionable because steroids have been used for long periods of time before the surgery.

Under these conditions, the operation is commonly performed in several stages. A standard ileostomy may be constructed to protect the anastomosis (Fig. 2). Alternatively, the proximal end of the rectum can be closed and placed back in the abdomen or brought out to the skin to drain as a "mucous fistula." Several months later, when the patient is fit and no longer taking steroids or immunosuppressive

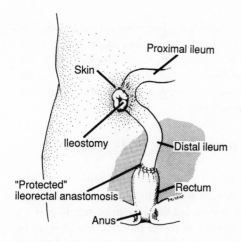

FIG. 2. When ileorectal anastomosis is performed in two stages, a temporary ileostomy is constructed to protect the anastomosis.

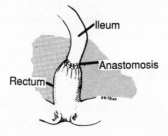

medications, the ileostomy can be closed and the ileum surgically connected to the rectum.

Patients usually stay in the hospital 8 to 12 days, and can resume normal activity 6 to 8 weeks later. Ileostomy closure requires a hospital stay of about 6 or 7 days.

COMPLICATIONS OF ILEORECTAL ANASTOMOSIS

Infection, e.g., abdominal or pelvic abscess, may occur in a small number of patients and is caused by leakage from the anastomosis. This may require reoperation to drain the abscess, although recent advances in needle aspiration and drainage under local anesthesia, using CT scanning guidance, have reduced the need for repeat surgery. In a study of 145 patients, leakage from the anastomosis occurred in only 3 patients. Reoperation for bowel obstruction caused by adhesions is also rare, as are pulmonary embolus (blood clot) and deep vein thrombosis. The risk of dying as a result of this operation is very small, and depends primarily on the severity of illness before surgery. Most recent studies, including the report of 145 patients, reported no mortality.

RETURN OF COLITIS SYMPTOMS

Continued inflammation of the rectum may occur. The more careful the surgeon is in selecting the proper candidate for this operation, the less likely it is that continued disease activity will be a problem. Conversely, the less selective the surgeon is in performing ileorectal anastomosis, the higher the failure rate will be. About 10% of well chosen patients will require subsequent proctectomy and ileostomy because of continued rectal inflammation.

BOWEL FUNCTION AFTER ILEORECTAL ANASTOMOSIS

After surgery, most people average four to five soft bowel movements per day. About 5% have bowel movements that awaken them at night. Incontinence or severe diarrhea may prompt removal of the rectum but this should be rare in patients properly chosen for this operation. The number of bowel movements can often be reduced by a series of exercises designed to stretch the rectum and train it to hold larger volumes of stool. Antidiarrheal medications such as Lomotil® or Imodium® are used by about 20% of patients. Intermittent rectal bleeding is treated with sulfasalazine or steroids given rectally or orally.

THE RISK OF CANCER

In a review of 17 series, only 3% of patients with ileorectal anastomosis developed cancer in the remaining rectum. The risk is related to the duration of the disease. The practice of periodic proctoscopy and mucosal biopsy should further lessen the incidence of such cancer. If dysplasia is found in the rectum at some time after surgery, a timely proctectomy (removal of the rectum) can be performed, followed by the construction of a standard ileostomy. Alternatively, the ileoanal anastomosis or the Kock pouch (continent ileostomy) could be performed.

PATIENT SATISFACTION

Clearly, satisfaction with the ileorectal anastomosis is directly related to good bowel function. Among those patients without active bowel disease, 96% were satisfied with the operation. Finally, in the event a patient with an ileorectal anastomosis requires further surgery, other options exist, including a standard ileostomy or a pelvic reservoir with ileoanal anastomosis or a Kock pouch.

27/ Ileoanal Anastomosis With or Without Reservoir

The ileoanal anastomosis is an operation for ulcerative colitis that removes all the diseased tissues, yet maintains the usual route of fecal elimination through the anal canal. Because the operation preserves intestinal continuity, no permanent ileostomy is required.

REASONS FOR PERFORMING THIS OPERATION

Ulcerative colitis is a disease that affects the inner lining of the large intestine without involving the underlying muscles. Thus, it is possible to remove all the disease without removing the entire colon, appendix, and lining of the rectum. While most of the abnormal colon is removed in its entirety, all but the inner lining of the rectum may be saved. After excising just the inner lining of the rectum, the surgeon can then pull the last part of the ileum through the remaining sleeve of rectum and attach it to the anus (Fig. 1). This operation thus leaves the muscles of the anal sphincter around the end of the rectum and anal canal intact. This provides a barrier against the accidental discharge of fecal contents through the anus. Also, the chance of damaging the nerves to the bladder and sex organs is minimized in this operation because the lining of the rectum is removed by operating through the anal opening itself and not through the nerve and other tissues around the rectum. Also, because no incisions are made on the outside of the rectum, there is no perineal wound.

Contraindications To This Operation

Individuals with ulcerative colitis are candidates for this operation, but those with Crohn's disease are not. This is because Crohn's disease frequently involves the small intestine, and what is normal small intestine at the time of surgery may become diseased at a later date. When recurrence occurs, complications such as fistulas, abscesses, and bleeding are likely. Moreover, subsequent operations might necessitate the loss of a significant amount of small intestine. Obviously, already diseased small intestine cannot be used for this anastomosis.

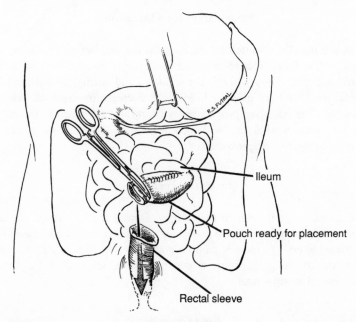

FIG. 1. Placement of the completed ileal pouch into the rectal sleeve, to be sutured to the anus.

Contraindications to this procedure also exist in those patients with ulcerative colitis. Those who are excessively obese are not candidates for this operation, because the excess fatty tissue limits the surgeon's ability to stretch small intestine to the anal canal to create the new rectum. Patients who have developed a cancer in the rectum as a consequence of their colitis are not candidates for the operation. In order to cure a rectal cancer, it is necessary to remove the entire rectum and anus; therefore, the ileoanal operation cannot be done. In contrast, ulcerative colitis patients who have developed cancer of the colon can still be considered for the anal anastomosis, provided the cancer can be excised completely at the time of operation.

Those with severe stricture or narrowing of the anal canal should not have this operation, because the new rectum cannot expand enough to accommodate the increased volumes of liquid stool common during the postoperative period. In addition, individuals who have sustained damage to the anal sphincter from previous disease or operations should not undergo the procedure, because they might not have a strong enough anal sphincter to hold back the increased volume of liquid stool after operation.

Preparation for Operation

Patients are usually admitted to the hospital the day before operation, and are placed on a clear liquid diet to decrease the amount of food bulk present in the gastrointestinal tract. They also receive laxatives and enemas to flush out the gastrointestinal tract, and are given antibiotics to decrease the bacterial count in the fecal material. The operative procedures are carefully explained to the patients so that they are aware of what they will encounter (*See Chapter 22 for a detailed discussion of preoperative preparation*).

Operative Technique

The operation is performed in two stages. During the first stage, the diseased colon and rectal lining are removed, the ileum is joined to the anal canal either in a straight (end to end) fashion or using a pouch created from adjacent loops of ileum. A *temporary* loop ileostomy is constructed, which is closed at the second operation several months later.

First Operation

The patient is placed in the face-up position with the legs apart. A vertical midline abdominal incision is made. The presence of ulcerative colitis is verified, and the existence of other abnormalities in the abdomen carefully noted.

Once the diagnosis is confirmed, the entire colon and the proximal rectum are removed; the distal rectum is stapled shut. In most cases, the ileum is connected to the rectum using a pouch made from the last 30 cm (12″) of ileum (see Fig. 1). Either sutures or staples can be used to make the pouch. The type of pouch made depends on the patient's individual anatomy and the preference of the surgeon. The surgeon may elect not to use a pouch at all, in which case the straight end of the ileum is sewn to the anal area. The surgeon uses the straight ileum when the small intestinal length is so short that a pouch would not reach the anal area. Use of the ileum alone without a pouch gives the most mobility and allows for the most distant reach. However, using the straight ileum means that in the early months and years after the operation, the patient will experience more diarrhea than occurs when a pouch is used. (Figure 2 illustrates the straight ileoanal anastomosis and the J and S pouches.)

Once the pouch is constructed, the surgeon begins operating through the anal opening and removes the innermost lining (mucosa) of the remaining rectum. The previously constructed ileal pouch (or straight ileum) is then brought down *within* the sleeve of remaining rectum and is joined to the anus.

In most cases, a temporary loop ileostomy is then created in the right lower quadrant of the abdomen. The ileostomy diverts intestinal contents away from the newly constructed pouch, allowing it to heal. This procedure decreases the possi-

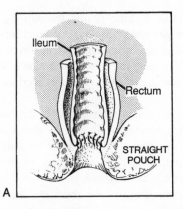

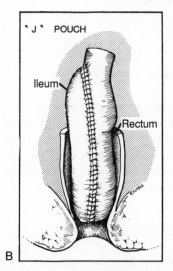

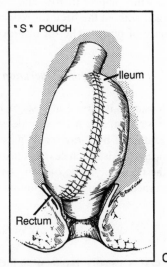

FIG. 2. Types of reservoir used with ileoanal anastomosis. **A**: The straight ileoanal anastomosis. **B**: The ileal "J" pouch-anal anastomosis. **C**: The ileal "S" pouch-anal anastomosis.

bility of a leak or an infection around the anastomosis. However, in cases where the dissection goes smoothly and the junction between the pouch and the anus is made without tension and with good blood supply, the operation can be done as a single-stage procedure without an ileostomy. If an ileostomy is used, it is usually closed at a second operation several months after the initial procedure.

Postoperative Course after First Operation

In the first few days after the first operation, the patient receives nothing by mouth and is fed intravenously. Pain medications (narcotic or nonnarcotic analgesics) are given by injection. A tube passed through the nose into the stomach keeps the stomach free of gas and fluid until intestinal function returns. The ileostomy usually begins to discharge intestinal contents on or about the fourth or fifth postoperative day, at which time the nasogastric tube can be removed and fluids can be taken by mouth. The diet is then gradually increased to include solids over the next 3 to 4 days.

Abdominal drainage tubes and a tube placed in the bladder at the time of the operation usually can be removed on about the fifth postoperative day. Patients are encouraged to sit up in a chair and may even be walking the day after operation. The hospital stay is usually between 10 and 14 days and shortly after discharge everyday activities can be resumed.

The most frequent complications of the operation are intestinal obstruction and infection, which appear in 10% and 5% of patients, respectively. Both can usually be managed without the need for reoperation, but reoperation is sometimes needed for drainage of pus or relief of obstruction.

Second Operation: Attaching the Pouch

The ileostomy is closed at a second operation performed about 2 months after the first operation. Just before the ileostomy is closed, the ileal pouch and anal canal are examined by x-ray techniques to ascertain that healing is complete. This second operation is much less extensive than the first. A small incision is made around the ileostomy. The opening (stoma) in the bowel is sewn closed, and the ileum returned to its usual position inside the abdomen.

Postoperative Course after Second Operation

Recovery is usually rapid after the second operation, although a nasogastric tube and intravenous feedings are given for 3 to 4 days until the bowels start to move. After bowel function has returned, a clear liquid diet is begun. At first, stools are frequent and liquid, but gradually thicken and decrease in number over the next few days. Bulking agents like Metamucil® and antidiarrheal medications such as Imodium® are useful in thickening the stool, slowing intestinal transit, and decreasing output. Most patients are ready for discharge on about the seventh postoperative day.

LONG-TERM RESULTS

Upon returning home, most people gradually increase their diet and activities, so that they are eating normally and have resumed their regular activities by 6 weeks after operation. The frequency of bowel movements gradually decreases with time. By 6 months after the operation, most people can expect approximately

5 soft, semiformed bowel movements during the day and 1 bowel movement at night. This pattern stays relatively constant. Continence is usually excellent, especially during the day. About 25%–30% of patients will have slight fecal spotting at night, i.e., a spot of fecal staining on a perineal pad once or twice a week during sleep. Fecal spotting also decreases with time, and virtually stops by 5 years after operation.

Sexual and urinary function are usually not affected by the surgery. Ninety-five percent of men report satisfactory sexual performance and potency. Although about 7% of women have painful intercourse once the surgical wounds have healed, nearly all women have normal sexual responses and are fertile. Most women who become pregnant after surgery are able to deliver vaginally. In general, the quality of life after recovery from the operation differs little from that of healthy people.

COMPLICATIONS OF THE ILEOANAL ANASTOMOSIS

In the weeks or months after the operation some patients may develop an inflammation in the pouch called "pouchitis." Symptoms of pouchitis include diarrhea, a small amount of blood in the stool, fever, nausea, and a general feeling of malaise. The exact cause of pouchitis is not known, but it may be related to the overgrowth of bacteria in the pouch. One thing is clear: pouchitis is *not* a recurrence of ulcerative colitis. Pouchitis usually can be treated with antibiotics such as metronidazole, which suppress bacterial growth. Response is usually prompt but pouchitis can reappear.

Absorption of most nutrients, minerals, and vitamins is normal after this operation. Patients are encouraged to try all types of foods, except perhaps natural laxatives, like prunes or grape juice. No cancers have appeared in the ileal pouches of persons followed for up to 15 years after operation. In rare cases, absorption of vitamin B12 is reduced and supplemental injections may be necessary.

28 // Continent Ileostomy

The continent ileostomy (Kock pouch), developed in Sweden by Dr. Nils Kock, represented an early alternative to standard ileostomy for ulcerative colitis patients who required colectomy. The advantage of the Kock pouch was that for the first time patients who had a total colectomy did not have to wear an external appliance to collect their intestinal wastes. Instead, an internal reservoir was created out of several loops of intestine which could be drained periodically by inserting a catheter through an abdominal stoma. At other times, the stoma was covered by a simple bandage.

WHO SHOULD HAVE THIS OPERATION?

The continent ileostomy is the operation of choice in patients with poor anal sphincter tone or a low-lying rectal malignancy. It is a preferable operation for those patients in whom the very thought of having frequent loose stools, perhaps with incontinence, is intolerable. It is also an option in a patient with failed ileoanal anastomosis, because the intestinal reservoir can be preserved and reused to construct the Kock pouch. Individuals with proctocolectomy and standard ileostomy requiring revision of the stoma might consider conversion to a continent ileostomy, as should those who cannot adjust to wearing an ileostomy appliance.

WHO SHOULD *NOT* HAVE A CONTINENT ILEOSTOMY?

There are several situations in which continent ileostomy cannot be constructed. In ulcerative colitis patients undergoing emergency proctocolectomy with toxic megacolon or massive hemorrhage, the additional time needed to construct the continent ileostomy is simply not justified. It is much safer to construct the reservoir ileostomy at a second stage, after the colon and rectum have been removed and the patient has been restored to good health. This construction of a continent ileostomy is also not justified in patients with Crohn's disease. If the disease were to recur in the small intestine (most likely in the surgically created pouch), the pouch would have to be removed, and with it up to 2 feet of invaluable small intestine needed for absorption of nutrients.

Most surgeons do not perform this operation in severely debilitated or malnourished individuals or in those suffering from severe side effects of steroid therapy. They also prefer not to construct a reservoir in cases where the rectum is left in after colectomy, because the presence of a reservoir in the pelvis can make it extremely difficult to remove the rectum when it becomes necessary in the future. In this case, it is wiser to perform a standard ileostomy, and, if the patient wishes, to convert to a continent ileostomy when the rectum is removed.

PERFORMING THE OPERATION

After removal of the diseased colon and rectum, approximately 18″ of terminal ileum are used to construct the reservoir and its components, the valve and outflow tract (Fig. 1). The surgeon then fashions a 1½″ to 2″ valve by turning the outflow tract back on itself and fixing it in place with a series of staples and/or sutures. The serosal surface of the ileum is abraded, which causes the reservoir to adhere to the abdominal wall and to prevent slippage of the valve. The surgeon must be careful to abrade the serosal surface just the right amount. Too much abrasion will result in a hole in the valve (valve fistula) or sloughing of the valve and outflow tract; too little will result in slippage of the valve. The use of a permanent synthetic device to hold the valve in place will reduce the tendency of the valve to slip, but will greatly increase the likelihood of a valve fistula. For these reasons, such devices are not used.

When the operation is finished, the stoma is at skin level and the patient wears just a small dressing to prevent soiling clothes with mucous discharge. After surgery, a catheter is left in the reservoir for about 3 weeks. The patient intubates

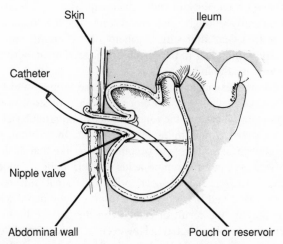

FIG. 1. A schematic diagram of the completed continent ileostomy, showing a catheter in place in the outflow tract.

(empties) the reservoir every 2 hours in the early postoperative period. The interval between intubations is gradually increased so that by 4 months after surgery the pouch is emptied approximately every 4 hours during the day and the patient can sleep through the night.

Increased intraabdominal pressure, as with exercise, coughing, or sneezing, is to be avoided unless the pouch has been emptied recently. Increased pressure and overfilling could cause the value to slip. Patients who develop upper respiratory infections during the first 4 to 6 months after surgery are instructed to tape the ileostomy catheter in place to avoid valve slippage during bouts of coughing and sneezing.

The individual with a continent ileostomy learns quickly that thick stool will prolong the emptying time to the point of annoyance and will require frequent insertions of the catheter to empty the pouch. In an effort to get thick stool to drain more quickly, some patients will press on the abdomen to increase intraabdominal pressure and hasten the drainage. This must be avoided because, once again, it increases the likelihood of valve slippage. At 1 year after surgery, you will spend 5 to 10 minutes 4 times a day emptying your reservoir. A minimum of two emptyings a day is necessary to reduce the risk of developing pouchitis, a subject to be discussed more fully later.

THE RESERVOIR AFTER SURGERY

The volume contained in the reservoir increases considerably after surgery. At the time of construction, the reservoir holds approximately 2 to 3 ounces. Although the final size of the reservoir varies depending on the frequency of intubation, most reservoirs eventually reach a volume of 1 pint. Those patients in whom the reservoir reaches a capacity of more than a quart are probably not emptying the reservoir frequently enough, and are risking the development of complications. During the first year after surgery, many of the sutures and staples used to construct the valve will appear in the pouch drainage. This is normal and does not mean that the valve is slipping.

All ileostomies are associated with changes in the number and type of bacteria found in the intestinal contents. The prolonged storage of stool in the reservoir of the continent ileostomy increases the total number of a particular class of bacteria, called anaerobic bacteria, found in the intestinal tract. In addition, the inner lining of the reservoir changes over time and becomes more like that of the colon. Nonetheless, electrolytes, sugars, and amino acids (protein building blocks) are all absorbed normally, However, there appear to be some small differences in the absorption of vitamin B12 and bile salts in the reservoir compared with the standard ileostomy. This may be the result of changes in the surface lining, or by the increased number of anaerobic bacteria. However, it is no more likely that serious metabolic imbalances will develop in those with the continent ileostomy than in those with the standard ileostomy.

EARLY COMPLICATIONS OF CONTINENT ILEOSTOMIES

Most of the early complications of this procedure are similar to those of any abdominal operation. However, there are a number that occur frequently and are related to the construction of the reservoir rather than to the proctocolectomy itself.

Suture Line Leak

Within the first week, suture line leaks or bleeding from suture lines will almost certainly need temporary diversion of intestinal contents with a temporary ileostomy to control infection and achieve healing. Suture line leaks, occurring from the 8th to the 20th day, usually respond quite well to tube drainage. Temporary diverting ileostomy is used only rarely. Suture line leaks are better prevented than treated, and can be avoided if the ileal reservoir is drained appropriately, and if the surgeon chooses patients who are not severely debilitated.

Destruction of the Outflow Tract

The outflow tract, that portion of ileum connecting the reservoir to the skin and including the nipple valve, may become necrotic if its blood supply is interfered with. This complication can occur if the nipple valve is too long, as occurs in very obese patients. If ischemic necrosis (death of tissue caused by insufficient blood flow) occurs there will be a large volume of leakage around the catheter with destruction of the stoma itself. The problem is best managed by keeping the reservoir empty with a special drainage system, enabling the outflow tract to shrink to the size of the catheter. It then can be revised surgically. Some surgeons use an ordinary baby pacifier to keep the tract in the abdominal wall open between intubations, and many patients have used this technique so successfully that they have been reluctant to have a surgical revision to correct the problem!

LATE COMPLICATIONS OF CONTINENT ILEOSTOMIES

Slippage of the Nipple Valve

This complication occurs most frequently in the first year after surgery and often results from waiting too long to empty the pouch during the first several months. If this occurs, you may begin having difficulty inserting the catheter and may notice some leakage of gas or stool from the stoma. At the first episode of difficult intubation, it is best to consult your surgeon, who will probably place a catheter in the reservoir and tape it securely in place for several weeks. If the slippage at this point has been minimal, the valve may fix in this new position with no further difficulty. As a rule, however, once significant slippage of the nipple valve has begun, an operation to revise the valve will be necessary.

Hole in the Nipple Valve (Valve Fistula)

Most episodes of leakage of stool and gas around the ileostomy catheter in the early postoperative period are caused by the catheter not being in proper position. If leakage continues after the catheter has been repositioned or removed, it is likely that a valve fisula has developed, a condition that can be verified by endoscopy or barium study of the pouch. Valves that have been reinforced with permanent foreign materials can develop fistulas years after surgery. Patients with nipple valve fistulas near the base of the valve generally require revisional surgery unless the opening is small enough to cause only minimal incontinence.

Skin Stricture

There are a number of patients who develop thick scars around the stoma which interfere with intubation. A skin stricture can also develop in patients in whom there has been sloughing of the outer portion of the stoma. This problem can often be managed by using a baby pacifier, without the need for further surgery. Most patients are somewhat reluctant to use a pacifier permanently, and surgery often becomes necessary. This can be done as an outpatient procedure using local anesthesia.

Prolapse of the Nipple Valve

Prolapse of an intact nipple valve occurs most often in patients who have had a previous operative revision of the valve. During the period of prolapse, the valve leaks gas and stool. The nipple valve is usually easily reduced and a catheter can be inserted without difficulty. Prolapse of the valve may also occur during strenuous exercise and occasionally during the last trimester of pregnancy. If you develop a prolapsed nipple valve during pregnancy, you will usually have no further difficulty once delivery has occurred. If repeated prolapse occurs, you will probably need revisional surgery.

Pouchitis (Inflammation of the Pouch)

Pouchitis causes diarrhea and bleeding in the reservoir, accompanied by a low-grade fever, malaise, and weight loss. Pouchitis can be diagnosed by endoscopy and your surgeon will try to exclude the possibility that you have recurrent Crohn's disease which was not apparent at the time of the initial procedure. Pouchitis is usually related to stasis, i.e., long intervals between intubations in the early postoperative period. There is a necessary phase of "mucosal adaptation" before the inner surface of the reservoir can tolerate prolonged periods between intubations. Most patients with pouchitis respond rapidly to "broad spectrum" antibiotics or antimicrobial agents such as metronidazole (Flagyl®), frequent intubations, and irrigation of the reservoir. The rapid response to antibiotics suggests that there is a significant overgrowth of bacteria that causes this inflammatory response.

In approximately 5% of patients, pouchitis will be recurrent and troublesome. It is in this group that an error in the original diagnosis is most likely. If you have more than one episode of pouchitis, it is wise to irrigate the pouch several times a week and increase the frequency of intubation in an effort to reduce the bacterial content in the reservoir.

Undiagnosed Crohn's Disease

Occasionally, a continent ileostomy is constructed inadvertently in a patient who has Crohn's disease and not ulcerative colitis. This can usually be avoided if the surgeon uses strict criteria when selecting candidates for the operation. If there is even the slightest suggestion that Crohn's disease may be present, this type of surgery should not be considered. Moreover, conversion from a standard ileostomy to a continent ileostomy should not be performed unless it is certain the patient does not have Crohn's disease.

Occasionally, however, when Crohn's disease occurs in the reservoir, an excellent response can be achieved with medical therapy. Steroids or metronidazole can be instilled directly into the reservoir or it can be irrigated with nonabsorbable antibiotics. It is also possible that 5-ASA enemas may help to reduce the inflammation. If the recurrence of Crohn's disease is in the segment of small intestine leading directly into the reservoir, it is often possible to resect the involved segment, leaving the reservoir intact. The best treatment, of course, is proper patient selection so that the problem does not arise in the first place.

SUCCESS WITH THE CONTINENT ILEOSTOMY

Surgeons stress that reliability and a cooperative attitude in their patients is of paramount importance to ensure a successful result with this operation. It is essential to perform intubation in the proper manner and to adhere to a rather rigid schedule early in the postoperative period. Before accepting a patient for the continent ileostomy, a surgeon will spend considerable time in the initial preoperative interview explaining the method of emptying the reservoir, and will often encourage the candidate to discuss the operation and its postoperative management with patients who have had a continent ileostomy.

RESULTS

In a study of 500 individuals with a continent ileostomy, complete control of gas and fecal discharge were achieved in 90% of those studies, 1 year after operation. Fifteen percent of these patients required some form of revisional surgery, usually for difficulty in intubation, but also for incontinence, prolapse, or skin stricture. Twenty percent of patients having one revision required further revisional surgery. It is interesting that most patients will elect to have multiple surgical revisions of their reservoirs rather than wear an external ileostomy appliance.

Revisional surgery is a procedure with low morbidity, since pouch-related reoperations are generally performed through incisions around the stoma. Even construction of a completely new nipple valve can be performed through this incision. The hospital stay is short, and rapid return to activity is the rule.

29 // Limited Colectomy

Ulcerative colitis begins in the rectum and later extends upward to involve the sigmoid colon and rest of the intestine. The natural history of ulcerative colitis is that with time, the entire colon may become involved. For this reason the operation of choice for ulcerative colitis has been removal of the entire colon and rectum (total proctocolectomy). The only exceptions to this have been the ileoanal and ileorectal anastomoses, in which minimally diseased rectum is used. Recently, some investigators have recommended performing a limited colectomy in which only the most severely involved part of the colon is removed.

PRESERVING THE RIGHT COLON

An operation in which the right (ascending) colon is retained has been performed in several centers, in a few highly selected patients with ulcerative colitis who were felt to have no disease in this segment of the colon, as determined either radiologically, by gross inspection, or by frozen section examination at the time of operation. The right colon is that portion of the large intestine that is best able to absorb fluid and electrolytes. The obvious benefit of preserving the right colon (with the ileocecal valve) is fewer and firmer bowel movements. Patients with colostomies at this level also have less trouble with dehydration and electrolyte imbalance and with stoma management than those with ileostomies who have a higher volume of output through the stoma.

In one series of 11 patients in whom the right colon was retained and a colostomy constructed, 10 were followed for an average of 10 years without evidence of recurrent disease. In another series of 6 patients who had preservation of the right colon with construction of a coloanal anastomosis (joining of the remaining colon to the anus), 5 of the 6 patients considered the operation acceptable after follow-up of more than 10 years. In this group of patients, biopsies showed inflammatory cells in the retained colon, but no evidence of ulceration. The significance of these findings is yet to be established.

Unfortunately, it is impossible to predict at the time of operation whether ulcerative colitis will extend to the transverse or right colon. If extension occurs and medical treatment cannot control symptoms, another operation may be necessary.

Chances of postoperative recurrence seem reduced when biopsies of the right colon are *normal* before surgery. However, because of the potential for a second operation, there is only a limited role for this approach in the surgical treatment of ulcerative colitis. Limited colectomy should only be employed when both patient and surgeon understand its risks and benefits.

Operations for Crohn's Disease

30 / Resection, Bypass, Proctocolectomy, and Other Surgical Options

Increased understanding of the natural history of Crohn's disease and its response to various treatments, including operation, has gradually changed the approach to its optimal surgical management. Since most (about 75%) patients with Crohn's disease will require an intestinal operation at some point in their lives, it is important for each patient to have a full understanding of what can and cannot be expected from this form of treatment. It has been learned and accepted by most authorities that, over time, the disease will recur after restorative (without external stoma) operation in most patients (about 75% within 15 years). Furthermore, increasing numbers of experts agree that taking out or bypassing longer segments of normal intestine upstream and downstream from the diseased intestine does nothing to improve this high rate of recurrence or to lengthen the time it takes for the recurrent disease to manifest itself. Thus, the goal of operation in Crohn's disease has gradually changed over the years from an attempt to "cure" and eradicate the disease completely to a strategy based on solving the problem or complication that brought the patient to operation. Moreover, this is done with an eye to conserving as much intestine as possible, at times leaving in segments that are diseased but functioning.

Patients and their physicians may be unduly optimistic about what operation can accomplish, or they may feel that there is no point in surgical treatment since the Crohn's disease eventually recurs after operation. Under the right circumstances, operation can be of enormous immediate and long-lasting benefit, especially when modern, conservative surgical strategy is employed. Based on these considerations, the indications for operation in Crohn's disease are those outlined in Chapter 19 and include: 1) failure of optimal medical treatment to allow the patient to function and be comfortable, 2) presence of intolerable side effects from the medications used to treat the disease, or 3) development of life-threatening complications of the disease process, such as abscess, intestinal obstruction, perforation, or bleeding.

Traditionally, two techniques have been used to deal with portions of the intestine that have been so severely damaged by Crohn's disease that one or more of the above indications for operation is present: resection (removal) of the diseased portion and bypass of the affected segment. When resection is done, the severed normal ends are usually joined unless there is severe infection or some other contraindication present, in which case a temporary ileostomy or colostomy may be necessary. In cases of colonic or rectal involvement or when the anal sphincters have been destroyed by fistulas, there will be no usable rectum and a permanent ileostomy or colostomy may be necessary. The choice of procedure for a given patient depends on the location and extent of the affected segment, and the severity of the disease and the type of complication present.

TECHNIQUE OF OPERATION

The location of the abdominal incision varies with the specific portion of intestine to be removed, the presence of any complications, and the preference and experience of the surgeon. It may be vertical or transverse. If the incision is vertical, it may be made on the right side, left side, or in the midline. In patients whose disease involves the colon, many surgeons avoid incisions impinging on the right lower portion of the abdomen since this is the best location for constructing an ileostomy which could become necessary at a later date or is planned as part of the procedure being done.

Once the abdomen is opened, all the abdominal organs are inspected and palpated as in any abdominal operation. Particular attention is given to the colon, small intestine, duodenum, and stomach to confirm and augment preoperative x-ray and endoscopic assessment of disease location, extent, and severity. The findings on exploration sometimes can call for modifications of the planned procedure. Modifications also may be necessary because of unforeseen circumstances that could arise during the operation, such as a change in the patient's condition.

RESECTION AND ANASTOMOSIS

In this procedure, the segment of intestine prompting surgery is removed (resected), dividing it from the remainder of the intestine. The two cut ends are then rejoined by sewing them together with suture material (anastomosis; Fig. 1). Over the years, considerable controversy has surrounded the question of how much healthy bowel should be removed on either side of the diseased segment. However, as explained earlier, there appears to be no point in removing long segments of undiseased intestine. Therefore, most surgeons divide the intestine rather close to the diseased segment(s) provided that the tissue appears healthy and will therefore hold the sutures and allow the anastomosis to heal.

Intestine that looks relatively healthy on the outside may be diseased inside, so once the resected segment of bowel is removed, it is examined immediately by a pathologist who inspects the inner or mucosal surface of the intestine. The pathologist and surgeon now determine how much disease is present and whether or not the surgical margins look healthy enough to be sutured. If not, another segment will be resected to ensure that the anastomosis will remain healthy and intact.

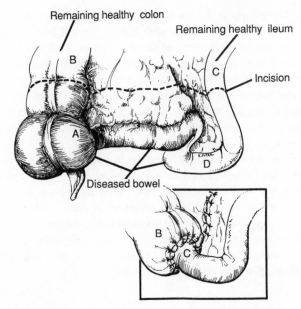

FIG. 1. Resection of diseased segment (A to D) with anastomosis of healthy ileum (C) to colon (B).

Depending on the specific portion of the gastrointestinal tract that is resected, the procedure is given various names. In general, the anatomic names for the two cut ends are abbreviated and the suffix "ostomy" is added to indicate that a communication now exists between the connected structures. For example, a procedure called "resection and ileoascending colostomy" would indicate that the ileum (ileo-) or last portion of the small intestine and the ascending colon (colo-) have been joined and are in communication with each other.

Occasionally, more than one segment of intestine requires surgical attention. As a general rule, it is safer to make one new connection in the intestine rather than two. However, unless the two diseased areas are very close to one another it is preferable to resect and rejoin each section rather than to remove a larger segment of bowel and thus sacrifice some healthy intestine. This is in harmony with the concept of conservative surgery.

BYPASS OPERATIONS

When bypass is carried out, the detour around the diseased intestine can be total (bypass with exclusion) or the diseased segment may merely be shortcircuited (nonexclusion bypass or bypass in continuity). Most surgeons prefer bypass with exclusion because it diverts (excludes) the intestinal contents from the diseased intestine, which presumably favors healing. Therefore, only bypass with exclusion will be described here. In this procedure the segment of intestine requiring bypass is identified as described above, and the intestine divided in a healthy area proximal (upstream from) and close to the diseased segment. The distal (downstream) end is sutured closed and the proximal end is then sutured to an opening made in the side of the intestine below the diseased portion, thus bypassing it. Typically the segment bypassed is the ileum and cecum and, in keeping with terminology explained above, this procedure is called an ileoascending or ileotransverse colostomy with exclusion.

In the past, many surgeons preferred exclusion bypass to resection and anastomosis because the former procedure was associated with fewer postoperative complications and had a lower mortality rate. With the advent of improved surgical and anesthetic techniques and better postsurgical care, both procedures are now performed with equal safety, barring special circumstances. Therefore, since complications including cancer, recurrence of disease, and perforation can occur in the bypassed segment, resection and anastomosis is the preferred procedure unless contraindications preclude its safe performance.

OPERATIONS FOR COLONIC CROHN'S DISEASE

Most patients with Crohn's disease involving the colon have ileal involvement as well (ileocolitis) and their surgical treatment is that described under resection and anastomosis. The same is true for those patients who have limited segmental involvement of the colon. However, there are some patients with extensive colonic disease, which involves the rectum as well, or whose sphincters are irreparably damaged who require a total removal of the colon and rectum (proctocolectomy).

Proctocolectomy is performed essentially as is described for ulcerative colitis (*See Chapter 25*), and any terminal ileum that is diseased is removed at the same time.

Unlike ulcerative colitis, colonic Crohn's disease does not always involve the rectum. In the 25% or more patients without rectal disease, it may be possible to resect only the abdominal portion of the colon and to connect the remaining portion of the ileum directly to the rectum, i.e., to perform a resection and ileoproctostomy or ileorectal anastomosis. (The performance of this procedure in ulcerative colitis is described at length in Chapter 26.) Although the rate of disease recurrence with ileorectal anastomosis is high, equalling that found with small bowel Crohn's disease, many patients may prefer to postpone, if even for a short time, the presence of an ileostomy and the accompanying changes in body function, physical appearance, and body image.

In previous years, some surgeons favored constructing a colostomy in the transverse colon in patients whose disease was confined to the descending colon and rectum. However, transverse colostomy with resection of the more distal colon presents no advantage over ileostomy and, over time, is usually followed by recurrence of Crohn's disease in the remaining colon. In the small minority of patients with Crohn's disease confined to the rectum, many will still elect to perform a sigmoid colostomy (external ostomy using the end of the sigmoid colon) with proctectomy (removal of the rectum).

After proctocolectomy for Crohn's disease, the rectal wound may heal slowly and then continue to drain, sometimes for several months or even years after removal of the rectum. This problem can frequently be avoided by suture of the rectal wound at the time of operation in suitable cases (*See Chapter 25*). If such an unhealed wound persists over a long period of time, it can be made to heal in the overwhelming majority of cases by remedial operation.

MAKING A DECISION FOR ILEOSTOMY IN CROHN'S DISEASE

Often the difficult decision to have an ileostomy in Crohn's disease results from consideration of many factors, including the failure of medical treatments, early recurrence after a first or second operation, and the desire to have an operation that allows a more normal life style. Despite the fact that colectomy and ileostomy *do not* preclude the possibility of disease recurrence, the incidence of recurrence in the ileostomy is significantly lower than after anastomotic procedures. Therefore, many patients in this situation choose life with an ostomy and the uncertainty of recurrence over repeated and continuous frustration with medical treatments. The following case presentation illustrates this point.

A 29-year-old woman had a 3-year history of Crohn's colitis unresponsive to treatment with sulfasalazine, prednisone, 6-MP, and metronidazole. Her small bowel was normal, but her colon was severely diseased from the cecum to the midportion of the sigmoid colon. Below the sigmoid, including the rectum and anus, her bowel was normal. A resection of the colon and anastomosis of the ileum to the sigmoid colon was advised. At the time of surgery, all obviously diseased bowel was removed, and the suggested ileosigmoidostomy was performed.

She remained well for a year and a half and then began to develop symptoms of intestinal obstruction that necessitated four hospitalizations within a period of 6 months. A barium enema showed a narrowed segment proximal to the site of anastomosis (Fig. 2) representing recurrent Crohn's disease. At flexible sigmoidoscopy, the remaining portion of the sigmoid colon, rectum, and anus remained normal, and the tight stricture at the anastomosis did not allow the sigmoidoscope to pass through.

This young woman did not wish to be placed on another course of prednisone, and it was felt that because of her symptoms and the tight stricture, that she should undergo resection of this recurrent disease and narrowed area. Because the remaining colon appeared normal, a resection and a reanastomosis of the bowel was suggested. Instead she chose to have an ileostomy. A resection of the diseased area was performed, the upper end of the sigmoid colon was closed off and

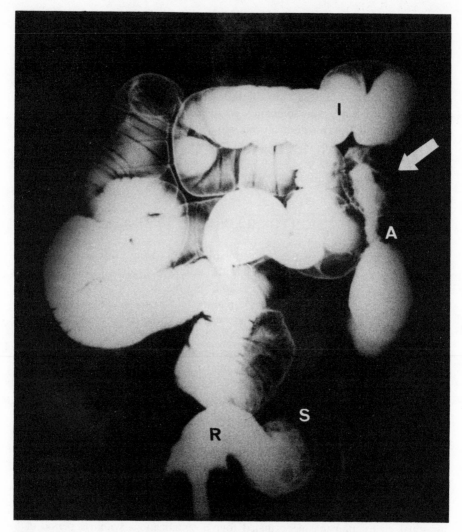

FIG. 2. Recurrent Crohn's disease (*narrowed area marked by arrow*) proximal to site of previous anastomosis (A). Adjacent structures are the ileum (I), sigmoid colon (S), and rectum (R).

left inside the abdominal cavity, and an ileostomy was fashioned in the right lower quadrant. She was taught to manage the stoma, and was discharged from the hospital within 10 days.

This case illustrates the example of a particular patient who did not wish to be exposed to the risk of having yet another recurrence after a second anastomosis and did not want any further drug therapy. She was quite convinced that despite the change in her body image, she would be better off having an ileostomy than having an early recurrence of her disease. This was the overriding consideration in her final decision. Her surgeon did not press the point but compromised with her and left the remaining part of her colon and rectum in place, should she decide at some point in the future to have the ileostomy taken down and connected again to her remaining colon.

The question of recurrence enters into the decision-making process every time an operation is considered for Crohn's disease. The last chapter in this section contains a full discussion of what is currently known about the likelihood of recurrence after surgery.

31 // Strictureplasty

The surgical approach to Crohn's disease has changed considerably during the half century or so since the disease was first described. Originally, surgeons believed that removal of the diseased intestine was curative. However, because of the high surgical mortality rate and the technical difficulty of performing resections at that time, surgical bypass of the involved bowel soon became preferable. Later, the pendulum swung back to radical removal of the disease when complications such as abscess, fistula, perforation, and cancer began to develop in the bypassed loops of bowel.

Today, a better understanding of the natural history of Crohn's disease has again altered the surgical approach. We now know that Crohn's disease can become active *anywhere* in the digestive tract from the mouth to the anus. More than one-half of patients have clinical involvement of both the small and large intestines (ileocolitis) at the time of diagnosis, and random biopsies from apparently normal bowel frequently reveal microscopic disease. What previously would have been called "recurrences" are probably activations of disease in new areas of intestine. Thus, we must accept that Crohn's disease *cannot* be cured by surgical removal and that the entire gastrointestinal tract is susceptible to intermittent activity and focal flare-ups throughout the patient's life.

Inherent in deciding which operation is most appropriate for a given patient with Crohn's disease is the understanding that he/she probably will have resurgence of disease activity that may require further operation. The possibility that extensive surgery may leave the patient insufficient length of intestine to absorb food makes it mandatory that the surgeon try to conserve as much bowel as possible.

Surgeons once thought that operations performed through diseased intestine frequently led to complications, or to early recurrence of Crohn's disease. Therefore, when removing a segment of bowel they frequently removed wide margins of healthy tissue adjacent to the diseased segment. Recent experience has shown that operations can be performed safely through diseased areas, and that removing large segments of disease does not prevent recurrence. Surgeons now remove only those segments of intestine that are responsible for the patient's problems. Thus, local removal of fistulas, abscesses, strictures, and perforated bowel has permitted

160

preservation of most of the intestine and resulted in an improved quality of life.

A natural extension of this "minimal surgery" philosophy in Crohn's disease is the application of a new operation called *strictureplasty* for narrowed areas (strictures) that cause intestinal obstruction.

Strictureplasty is the operative correction or widening of an intestinal narrowing without removal of bowel. Since strictures are often multiple and can involve long or widely separated parts of the bowel, this method of relieving obstruction is an attractive alternative to resection. The actual technique is a very old one but had not been used in IBD because surgeons feared the consequences of operating through diseased bowel. Since the early 1980s, strictureplasty has been used increasingly in the "minimal surgery" management of Crohn's disease.

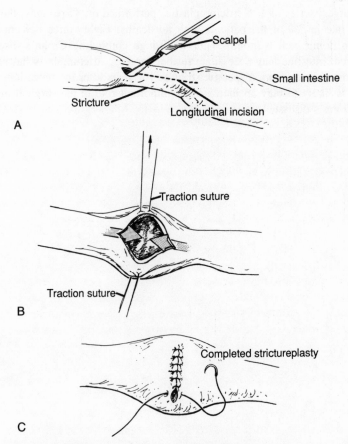

FIG. 1. A: In strictureplasty, the stricture is incised longitudinally into the lumen of intestine. **B:** Traction sutures are used to convert the longitudinal incision to a transverse one. **C:** Transverse incision is closed with one layer of interrupted sutures.

SURGICAL TECHNIQUE

Strictureplasty can be performed alone or in combination with other procedures. When done for a short stricture (Fig. 1), the narrowed segment of bowel is cut longitudinally and closed transversely, thus widening the narrowed area. For longer strictures, a more complicated closure is used. Some surgeons attempt to identify and correct all significant strictures in a single operation, even those that are not producing obvious clinical obstruction. At operation, a small balloon on a catheter is passed up and down the small intestine and wherever the balloon "hangs up," a strictureplasty is performed. Complications have been minimal and symptoms of obstruction have been alleviated considerably. As many as 16 strictureplasties have been performed at one operation, and strictureplasties have been combined with multiple resections and with balloon dilations of the small intestine (*See Chapter 32*).

In the largest series of 106 strictureplasties performed on 37 patients, there was a leakage rate in 7% of the patients with no deaths. Eighty-three percent of patients were doing well 6 months later. Although continuing Crohn's disease in other areas of intestine may necessitate further surgery, strictureplasty has relieved the symptoms arising from a specific stricture for years after the procedure. Strictureplasty is likely to play an increasingly important role in the surgical management of Crohn's disease.

32 / Endoscopic Dilation of Strictures

Procedures performed through the endoscope are becoming attractive alternatives in an attempt to avoid surgery and limit the extent of intestinal resections in Crohn's disease. When an area of bowel becomes so narrowed that it obstructs the flow of intestinal contents, removal of the strictured segment is the standard surgical approach. The preceding chapter describes strictureplasty as a means of conserving bowel in patients with many narrowed areas or in those who have previously had a substantial amount of intestine removed.

Recently, endoscopic techniques have been developed to dilate these chronic intestinal strictures. Although these techniques are not yet in general practice, they represent another option for the accomplished endoscopist to help a patient to postpone or avoid surgery or limit the amount of intestine that must be removed. Obviously, endoscopic dilation of a stricture may be attempted only if the narrowed area is within reach of the endoscope. The last part of the duodenum and the ascending colon or perhaps the terminal ileum are the usual limits of reach for the endoscope passed by mouth or rectum, respectively. Deeper areas of intestine may be reached if a resection has been performed previously or if the endoscope is passed during operation. This is accomplished when the surgeon introduces the endoscope into the intestine either by "feeding" bowel over it or passing it through a tiny incision in the bowel. Once the endoscope has reached the strictured area (Fig. 1A), a balloon catheter is passed through the endoscope and into the narrowed segment (Fig. 1B). The balloon is then inflated (Fig. 1C), thus dilating the stricture (Fig. 1D). The maximum diameter to which the stricture may be safely dilated is determined either by fluoroscopic monitoring during the procedure or simply by the endoscopist's clinical judgment; one convenient criterion is whether the endoscope will pass through a segment of bowel that did not allow it to pass before dilation.

Only a limited number of these transendoscopic balloon dilations have been performed in patients with Crohn's disease and follow-up has been rather short-term. The procedure appears to be painless and relatively safe, although the strictured area tends to narrow again after several months. Which strictures are best treated in this manner and whether the activity or chronicity of the disease influences the outcome of balloon dilation are yet to be determined.

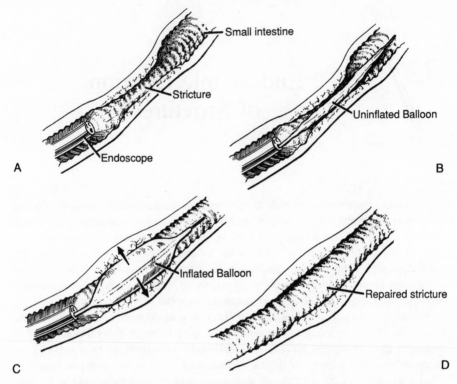

FIG. 1. A: Endoscope positioned at stricture. **B:** Deflated balloon catheter passed through the endoscope and positioned within the strictured area. **C:** Inflated balloon, dilating the stricture. **D:** Dilation complete, endoscope withdrawn.

33 // Operations for Perforations, Abscesses, and Fistulas

Because Crohn's disease may affect any part of the gastrointestinal tract, and because it has a tendency to recur after resection, surgeons are reluctant to operate unless a patient fails to respond to medical therapy or develops specific complications. Surgical intervention is often deferred until major complications occur. Complications may be subdivided into two varieties: "perforating" and "nonperforating." Nonperforating complications of Crohn's disease, including intestinal obstruction, hemorrhage, and toxic megacolon, have been covered in a previous chapter.

PERFORATING COMPLICATIONS

A perforation is a rupture of the gastrointestinal tract into the abdominal or peritoneal cavity. There are two types of perforating complications in Crohn's disease: abscess and fistula. An abscess is a localized collection of infected material, usually consisting of pus, intestinal contents, and bacteria. Abscesses may occur anywhere in the abdomen: between loops of bowel, under the diaphragm, in the pelvis, in the area behind the back lining of the abdominal cavity known as the retroperitoneum, or even within organs such as the liver or spleen. A fistula is a channel or tract between two or more organs. Fistulas may become lined with epithelial tissue and allow intestinal contents to pass from one organ to the other. Thus an ileovesical fistula allows stool or air to pass from the ileum into the bladder, while a rectovaginal fistula permits intestinal contents to pass into the vagina.

Although these complications represent serious developments in the course of Crohn's disease, they may be treated effectively provided they are well understood and promptly recognized. They are the natural outcome of a transmural disease, i.e., affecting all layers of the bowel wall. Fissures (cracks) may travel the full thickness of the bowel wall to perforate freely into the peritoneal cavity; alternatively, tracts may form abscesses between contiguous organs, or extend as fistulas directly into adjacent structures.

Symptoms of Perforation

Free or direct perforation into the peritoneal cavity results in sudden and severe abdominal pain, rigid abdominal muscles, shock, high fever, and sepsis (bacteria found in the blood stream). This toxic state is known as generalized peritonitis.

A perforation that has been contained by forming an abscess is characterized by a slower progression of the infection. Patients with contained perforations typically experience fever and a localized tenderness often with a palpable abdominal mass that represents the abscess. Such a mass can be felt by your physician during a careful examination of the abdomen and confirmed by x-ray, ultrasound, or CT examinations.

Fistulas may pass from one loop of bowel to another or from the intestinal tract to the surface of the body, often through the site of previous surgical incisions. Chronic skin irritation and infection may result.

SURGICAL TREATMENT

Direct perforation with peritonitis requires immediate surgery. Intraabdominal abscesses frequently require surgical drainage or resection although occasionally other nonsurgical treatments, including antibiotics and needle aspiration, may be successful. Abdominal fistulas may require surgery depending on their location and the patient's symptoms. Although many patients with fistulas are treated medically with various combinations of antibiotics, steroids, hyperalimentation, metronidazole, or 6-MP, most ultimately require surgical treatment.

Free Perforation

Free perforation is an acute problem that used to be a fatal complication of Crohn's disease but that today has a far better prognosis. Most free perforations occur in the distal ileum but no area of small or large bowel is spared this complication. At surgery, the segment of perforated bowel is removed and the remaining ends of bowel reconnected. The fecal stream is usually diverted from this connection (anastomosis) by a loop ileostomy. Once the bowel has healed, the ileostomy is taken down, allowing stool to flow normally.

Intraabdominal Abscess

Early and complete drainage of intraabdominal abscesses is the key to successful management of this serious complication. The surgeon usually drains the abscess using an abdominal incision, although alternate methods have been proposed. One such method involves introducing a long thin needle or catheter into the abscess cavity through the skin (percutaneous needle aspiration). The value of this method in treating intestinal abscesses is less established than its use with abscesses elsewhere because the underlying bowel disease that resulted in the abscess is left intact. In some instances, removal of the diseased bowel communicating with the abscess may be performed at the same time as incision and drainage of the abscess. In other cases, a resection is more safely performed at a second operation. If the two procedures, drainage and resection with anastomosis, are performed during one operation, proximal diversion of the fecal stream is advisable, especially in the ill or debilitated patient in whom wound healing will be delayed. Each abscess should be carefully evaluated and localized by x-ray examination, sonography, or CT scan before surgery.

Certain specific abscesses require special treatment. For example, a pelvic abscess that extends into the rectum can be drained directly through the rectum without the danger of contaminating the peritoneal cavity, thus eliminating the risk of spreading the infection into other areas of the body. Treatment of abscesses requires careful localization, meticulous surgical technique, and adequate drainage.

Fistulas

The surgical management of fistulas often requires that multiple areas of intestine be removed and a temporary diverting ileostomy be used to protect the anastomosis. With careful preoperative evaluation, bowel cleansing, and appropriate use of antibiotics, few complications can be expected.

When a fistula originates from severely diseased bowel, the segment of bowel usually must be removed along with the fistula. A fistula arising from relatively healthy bowel may occasionally be removed without the need for bowel resection. Rectovaginal fistulas still remain the most difficult fistulas to cure. These fistulas may be closed successfully in some patients with relatively localized rectal disease; medical therapy with metronidazole or 6-MP often leads to improvement (*See Chapters 7 and 10*).

34 // Perineal Operations

Crohn's disease may affect the rectum, anus, and perineum, causing painful abscesses, ulcers, and draining fistulas. Occasionally, perineal involvement may be the sole or initial manifestation of Crohn's disease, occurring commonly when there is disease in the lower colon. Typically, anorectal Crohn's disease can be the major reason for ill health and discomfort at a time when the bowel disease is quiet.

Although the reason why the disease affects the anorectum is unknown, Crohn's disease does attack areas of the bowel that contain lymphoid tissue. It is possible that through an immunologic or bacteriologic mechanism, the pockets of lymphocytes found in the lower rectum may hold a clue to the cause of these complications. Diarrhea caused by Crohn's disease probably contributes little to infections, which occur deep within the perirectal tissues. In fact, some patients with colostomies and ileostomies still have progressive and continuing perirectal infections, even after diversion of the fecal stream. Consequently, if an ileostomy or colostomy can be avoided, local operative therapy is the preferred treatment. Since disease of the upper and lower bowel and anorectal Crohn's disease often behave independently of one another, successful treatment of Crohn's disease in the small intestine or colon should not necessarily be expected to improve the anorectal situation.

TREATMENT STRATEGY

Any treatment strategy for the anorectal complications of Crohn's disease should emphasize relief of symptoms such as local pain, discharge, constipation, incontinence, and bleeding. In most instances, rectal pain is caused by an incompletely drained rectal abscess. If an abscess is difficult to locate, often because rectal examination is too painful, examination under anesthesia may be necessary. Fissures and hemorrhoids are rarely a cause of pain in patients with Crohn's disease.

Profuse discharge from the rectum is usually caused by one or more abscesses draining from a single fistula or many fistulas. Constipation may result from a stricture in the rectum, caused by scarring from a chronic rectal abscess or the disease itself. Incontinence, the inability to control bowel movements, may be the result of inappropriate rectal surgery or a persistent rectal infection that destroys the anal sphincter muscles. Rectal bleeding in Crohn's disease is usually a result of inflammation in the lower colon and/or rectum, but may be caused by hemorrhoids. Skin tags are flaps of skin around the anus that are caused by inflammation in people with Crohn's disease and that may be confused with large external hemorrhoids.

Any of these perineal expressions of Crohn's disease might cause you to seek surgical treatment. A knowledgeable surgeon approaches each of these complications individually and with great care, because of the tendency of surgical wounds in this area to heal poorly in the person with Crohn's disease. The reason for this poor healing is not well understood, but the use of medications such as metronidazole or 6-MP may speed up the healing process. In any case, judicious, well-timed surgery together with medical therapy may alleviate many of the symptoms of perineal Crohn's disease.

Treatment of Painless Perianal Complications

Skin tags are among the most common painless conditions associated with Crohn's disease. In general, they should not be removed because of their tendency to heal poorly. Most people who develop skin tags consider them unsightly and annoying, since they make it difficult to clean the perirectal area after bowel movements. However, after removal of the skin tags, ulcers may develop that can produce far greater problems than the skin tags themselves. Therefore the best course of action in treating skin tags is to avoid surgery unless absolutely necessary.

Painless anal fissures and fistulas usually do not require surgical treatment and often respond best to a course of metronidazole or 6-MP (*See Chapters 6 and 7*). A fistula that is adequately drained will ooze small amounts of material and usually will not cause any pain or discomfort. A rectovaginal fistula, however, is difficult to tolerate physically, psychologically, and sexually. If fecal discharge from the vagina is minimal, medical therapy may be successful and surgery should be delayed. If it becomes necessary, surgical repair of the rectovaginal fistula will be successful if the mucosal lining of the rectum is not badly ulcerated, inflamed, or scarred by Crohn's disease. More commonly, the surgeon may construct a temporary or permanent ileostomy or colostomy, depending on the condition of the rectum, and will repair the rectovaginal fistula or let it heal spontaneously. Recently, some surgeons have experimented with the use of gracilis muscle or inferior gluteal musculofascial flaps to correct rectovaginal fistulas.

Anal incontinence in the patient with anorectal Crohn's disease is usually the result of previous operations in this area. Direct surgical repair of the anal sphincter muscles may be complicated by the presence of perirectal infections and fistulas. In cases of anal incontinence, a thin stainless steel Thiersch wire may be wrapped around the lower rectum to act as a mechanical barrier to stool loss. Gracilis muscle transposition may also be appropriate in this situation, but its use is still experimental. Occasionally, a course of medical therapy may clear up the infection sufficiently to permit surgical correction.

Anorectal strictures are often caused by chronic abscesses in the soft tissues adjacent to the rectum, which may have been drained incompletely. The surgical approach involves drainage of this presumed abscess by a partial removal of the internal anal sphincter muscle. After this procedure the stricture usually can be opened by simple dilation.

When painless rectal bleeding occurs, it may not be possible to determine whether the bleeding is caused by hemorrhoids or by inflammation of the rectal mucosa. Under these circumstances, simple measures such as hemorrhoid injection sclerotherapy, rubberband ligation, or infrared photocoagulation may be beneficial. Protrusion through the anus of internal hemorrhoids also can be treated with these measures.

Treatment of Painful Perineal Complications

In Crohn's disease, pain in the perianal area is most often the result of a rectal abscess. A rectal abscess that occurs for the first time usually can be treated with simple incision and drainage. An abscess that develops between the muscles of the anus is treated by means of a partial internal anal sphincterectomy, in which part of the internal sphincter muscle is removed and the abscess unroofed. Fistulas resulting from the abscess then heal spontaneously. The concept that perirectal abscesses develop from intersphincteric abscess has particular applicability to the patient with Crohn's disease. Small incisions in the rectum are used, thus avoiding the problem of the unhealed perirectal wound. By restricting the excision to the internal sphincter and avoiding incisions in the external sphincter muscle, interference with anal continence is minimized. Even partial incontinence in a person with Crohn's disease who already has diarrhea is a dreaded complication that must be avoided. In one study of more than 300 patients with rectal abscesses who were treated in this manner, there were no cases of anal incontinence and fistulas healed in 85% of subjects. The surgeons using this approach were able to alleviate pain, allow the patient to function normally, and avoid recurrent abscess formation.

The patient with persistent undrained abscesses is likely to have difficulty with incontinence, stricture formation, or persistent sepsis. A conservative approach to surgery should not deprive a patient of a necessary operation. Appropriate perineal surgery can greatly improve the quality of life in individuals with anorectal Crohn's disease.

35 / The Question of Recurrence after Surgery

Since surgery does not cure Crohn's disease, but may be necessary at some point for two-thirds to three-quarters of persons with the disease, the question of recurrence is an important and troubling one. Long-term studies of patients operated on for Crohn's disease at major medical centers have shown that at least 75% to 80% of them will ultimately experience a recurrence. Does this mean that every person with Crohn's disease is doomed to a never-ending cycle of repeated operations and recurrences?

THE DEFINITION OF A RECURRENCE

There are some differences in the way people define this term. At one end of the spectrum, some investigators define a recurrence as any evidence at all that there is still some inflammation detectable anywhere in the intestine. By this definition, recurrence of Crohn's disease after surgery is virtually universal and almost immediate. For example, if all patients were to be subjected to colonoscopic examinations within a few months after surgery for Crohn's disease, whether or not they were having symptoms, 80% to 90% of them would have small pinpoint ulcerations characteristic of the disease in the area of the anastomosis. But if we look hard enough, these tiny ulcerations and other signs of inflammation often can be detected anywhere in the digestive tract, from mouth to anus, of just about anyone with Crohn's disease. Since, according to this view, the disease is always present in some subtle form everywhere throughout the intestinal tract, we should not speak of "recurrence" of a disease that has never been eradicated, but should instead refer only to "recrudescence" of a disease that is always potentially active. What is important to remember, however, is that microscopic abnormalities or changes seen through the endoscope do not always mean that symptoms will return.

At the other end of the spectrum, a recurrence could be defined as disease severe enough to require a second operation. Using this strict definition, recurrence rates are much lower, perhaps only 25% to 30% after 10 years and 40% to 50% after 20 years. Obviously, not all recurrent Crohn's disease is severe enough to require operation, so a "clinical" definition of recurrence must be used if we are concerned with the frequency of recurrent symptoms. By this definition, any return of symptoms, e.g., pain, diarrhea, fever, or weight loss, would be considered a recurrence if the symptoms could be shown to be caused by Crohn's disease. From this "middle-of-the-spectrum" viewpoint, the overall rates of postoperative recurrence are in the range of 20% by 2 years, 30% by 3 years, and about 40% to 50% by 5 years.

WHO IS LIKELY TO HAVE A RECURRENCE?

It is important to realize that all cases of Crohn's disease are not the same, nor are all operations for Crohn's disease alike. Many different factors have been implicated by different researchers as being important in determining postoperative recurrence rates. The biggest difficulty in trying to determine which of these variables are or are not important is that they may be interrelated. For example, the age of a patient at the time of surgery has something to do with how long he or she has had the disease, which in turn has something to do with the kind of complication that is requiring surgery. These factors may depend on the anatomic distribution of the disease, which in turn influences the choice of operative procedure. As a result, it is quite difficult to sort out which of these factors may be the important ones influencing recurrence.

One factor that seems to make a significant difference in most studies is whether the operative procedure itself entails a reanastomosis (reconnection) of intestines after removal of most of the colon, as opposed to an ileostomy. Neither form of operation offers any guarantee against postoperative disease recurrence, but most studies have suggested that the recurrence rates are only about one-third as great after ileostomy as after reanastomosis. Most people, however, still prefer to preserve intestinal continuity, even when they know that they risk a higher rate of recurrence.

A second factor influencing recurrence rates seems to be the "behavior pattern" of Crohn's disease. In some instances of Crohn's disease, for example, surgery becomes necessary only after many years of disease, usually as a result of progressive, insidious scarring leading to repeated episodes of partial obstruction or "blockages." In such cases, the *probabilities* favor a prolonged postoperative remission; recurrences often do not develop for 8 to 10 years. Note that we emphasize the concept of *probability*, since we are speaking here only of a trend—a statistical tendency among a certain group of patients—and nothing approaching a definite prediction for any one individual.

In sharp contrast are the more "aggressive" cases of Crohn's disease that rapidly ulcerate through the bowel wall, developing fistulas and abscesses within only a year or two from the initial onset of disease. In these circumstances, surgery is often unavoidable. The tendency, however, is for postoperative recurrences to appear more rapidly in these aggressive cases than they do in the more indolent cases of slowly developing obstruction, sometimes within 1 to 2 years after surgery. Once again, it is important to remember that these are general tendencies; individuals vary greatly, and, in fact, different studies of these trends have yielded differing results.

THE OUTCOME OF A RECURRENCE

Postoperative recurrence of Crohn's disease is almost invariably located at the site of anastomosis, where the remaining ends of relatively normal intestine have been reconnected. When the original disease is in the small intestine alone, the recurrence is usually situated on the small bowel side of the anastomosis. When the original disease is Crohn's colitis or ileocolitis, the recurrence may take place on either the small bowel side, the large bowel side, or both. In cases of ileostomy, the recurrences, when they do develop, are nearly always located at the end of the small bowel right up to and including the ileostomy itself.

Some recurrences affect only very short segments of intestine, perhaps as little as an inch or two. Others may extend for many feet up and down the intestinal tract. There is no clear basis for predicting which pattern might occur in any given case, but once a recurrence has taken place, there is usually no further spread beyond those points in the absence of further surgery. In other words, recurrent inflammatory disease in particular sections of bowel may wax and wane in intensity, but will rarely spread to other sections of bowel. There is a rough tendency for the clinical behavior of the recurrent disease to mimic the pattern that the original disease manifested before surgery (e.g., for obstructing disease ultimately to start reobstructing, for fistulous or abscess-forming disease to begin forming fistulas or abscesses again).

Another general characteristic of recurrent Crohn's disease after surgery is that it often proves more responsive to medical therapy than did the original preoperative disease. Only about 40% to 50% of patients with symptomatic recurrence after their first operation ever require a second operation for Crohn's disease during their lifetimes. Although we have all heard stories of unfortunate patients undergoing three, four, or even more operations for repeated recurrences, such cases constitute only a small fraction of patients who have surgery for Crohn's disease. Two of the largest studies of this problem have both arrived at the nearly identical figure of only 11% for the proportion of Crohn's disease patients undergoing one operation who will ever in their lives require a total of three or more operations.

WHAT CAN BE DONE TO PREVENT A RECURRENCE?

In a word: nothing. Neither meticulous surgical technique nor radical resections, neither strict diets nor preventive medications after surgery have been found to influence the rates of postoperative recurrence. New research studies of various medications are underway in the hope that they might reduce recurrence rates, but as of today, no amount of wishful thinking, careful eating, or clean living is believed to alter the risk of recurrent disease.

How Does This Affect the Decision to Have Surgery?

No one should have an operation if it is not necessary. The reluctance for surgery is understandably even greater when the odds are against the procedure being permanently curative. Nevertheless, most people with Crohn's disease will at some point have to undergo an operation for good and proper reasons: obstruction, fisulas and abscesses, hemorrhage, perforation, tumors, retarded growth and development, chronic disability, intolerable quality of life, etc. The overwhelming majority of these patients—even if they have suffered a recurrence along the way—view their quality of life and their degree of psychosocial function as having been improved by the operation.

Operation for Crohn's disease should be undertaken with careful consideration but without fear. Some patients may never experience a recurrence; for those who do, the recurrence may produce no major symptoms; even in cases with major symptoms, the disease may respond to medical treatment better than it did before surgery. The odds are somewhat against needing a second operation and greatly against needing a third.

Moreover, the period of remission after surgery, whether it is 1 year or 20 years, should be viewed as an opportunity to get on with life. The primary object of treating Crohn's disease, after all, is not simply to avoid surgery; it is to feel well, to function, and to enjoy life. If surgery can help to achieve these goals, then it should be faced without excessive or paralyzing anxiety about the question of recurrence.

PART 6

Special Surgical Situations

36 // Surgery and Pregnancy

The medical treatment of IBD during pregnancy and the influence of IBD and pregnancy on one another have already been discussed in Chapter 13. In this chapter we will consider the effects of pregnancy and delivery on a patient who has had surgery for IBD, and the effects of surgery on the pregnant patient. In brief, in the woman who has already had surgery and is doing well, pregnancy and delivery usually progress without additional problems caused by the IBD. On the other hand, complications of IBD that require an operation during pregnancy carry very serious implications for both mother and child; fortunately, the need for surgery during pregnancy arises very rarely.

As detailed in Chapter 13, it is generally believed that pregnancy has little influence on disease activity in Crohn's disease or ulcerative colitis. Women in remission at the beginning of pregnancy are likely to remain well throughout pregnancy; those who are ill at the time of conception will probably continue to have problems and are less likely to have a normal full-term delivery. Obviously, it is advantageous for both mother and baby that the pregnancy be delayed until the IBD is in remission. Sulfasalazine or corticosteroids can be used safely during pregnancy and are not thought to be harmful to the fetus. However, it is a good idea to postpone pregnancy if medical treatment is unsuccessful and the need for surgery seems imminent.

PREGNANCY AND DELIVERY AFTER OPERATION FOR IBD

After Ileostomy

In women who have had a colectomy and ileostomy for ulcerative colitis or Crohn's disease of the colon, relatively few ileostomy-related problems arise during pregnancy. A normal vaginal delivery can be expected without any additional complications caused by the surgery. Contrary to a common misconception, caesarean section should *not* be necessary in the woman with an ileostomy unless indicated for purely obstetrical reasons. Most obstetricians now feel that vaginal delivery is not only possible, but preferable. Successful pregnancy and delivery have been reported after a variety of operations for IBD, including ileorectal anastomosis, ileoanal anastomosis, and continent ileostomy (Kock pouch).

Obviously, the abdomen swells during pregnancy and softening and enlargement of many anatomical structures takes place. Thus, the position, contour, and size of the ileostomy change during pregnancy and may cause difficulty maintaining a good seal of the appliance around the stoma. A larger appliance may be needed and it may be impossible to use a belt. Many patients already use semi-disposable, lightweight appliances and customarily frame the faceplate with tape instead of relying on belts. In these patients, any adaptations and modifications necessary during pregnancy would be almost routine. Women who are not already familiar with these appliances and techniques will find that they are relatively easy to learn and adapt for pregnancy.

Occasionally, the ileostomy may prolapse because of the combination of enlargement and softening of the stoma together with the increase in intraabdominal pressure. If prolapse occurs, it is usually minor and of little consequence. To lessen the likelihood of prolapse, it is a good idea to avoid the use of a belt, which produces increased pressure on the thinned abdominal wall around the ileostomy. Using a soft pad (e.g., a portion of sanitary napkin or a cotton ball over the ileostomy) under a relatively loose elastic garment or band may be of some help. Awareness of this problem may help to prevent a major prolapse (one that does not reduce promptly after lying down and removal of the appliance)—a rare complication that requires prompt medical attention. Fortunately, the tendency to prolapse disappears quickly after childbirth.

Toward the end of pregnancy when the uterus becomes very large, it may displace and distort the ileostomy or adherent loops of intestine, causing partial or total intestinal obstruction. When this happens, it may be necessary to induce labor earlier than usual.

After Resection

After resection or bypass for Crohn's disease, pregnancy and delivery usually proceed normally, especially in women who are healthy. The fact that a previous operation has been performed has little effect on the outcome of pregnancy, although there may be a slightly increased tendency toward prematurity and spontaneous abortion.

The tendency of some women with Crohn's disease to develop perineal abscesses and fistulas will influence the advisability of vaginal delivery with episiotomy. In general, perineal complications occur most often when there is Crohn's disease of the colon and rectum. In women without perineal fistulas and abscesses, the more upstream from the rectum the Crohn's disease, the less concern there need be about vaginal delivery and episiotomy. Conversely, caesarean delivery should be strongly considered in women with severe perineal disease.

OPERATION DURING PREGNANCY

Operation for any condition during pregnancy raises many issues relating to the welfare of the mother and fetus. First of all, it is more difficult for the physician to make an accurate diagnosis of acute intraabdominal conditions in the pregnant woman. Confusion with the usual aches and pains of pregnancy may delay the realization that something is wrong. It is not uncommon for the abdominal cramps of a Crohn's disease flare-up to be confused with premature labor and vice versa; the distinction can be difficult even for the most experienced physician. The interpretation of the abdominal examination is also made more difficult because of displacement of inflamed intestine by the pregnant uterus. Moreover, normal pregnant women tend to be anemic and have an elevated white blood cell count so that these laboratory tests may be harder to interpret and less useful than in women with IBD who are not pregnant. Certain diagnostic procedures, such as x-ray studies, are helpful in the diagnosis of acute abdominal conditions but may be hazardous to the normal development of the fetus, especially in the first trimester of pregnancy.

Premature labor may be induced by any acute inflammatory process in the abdomen, by anesthesia, or by the manipulation entailed in an abdominal operation. In addition, anesthetic agents may pose hazards for the developing fetus. Operation, childbirth, and IBD *all* have a tendency to promote blood clotting, so that the three occurring together pose an increased risk of thrombophlebitis and pulmonary embolism (blood clots that travel to the lungs).

Because of these hazards to mother and fetus, physicians are hesitant to recommend diagnostic studies or surgery in their pregnant patients. Understandably, women, too, are reluctant to accept recommendations for diagnostic procedures and surgery, thus adding further to the dangers. Probably, more errors of omission than commission are made because both patient and physician are reluctant to pursue diagnosis and treatment of abdominal complaints during a pregnancy.

COMPLICATIONS OF ULCERATIVE COLITIS AND CROHN'S COLITIS

Every complication of colonic IBD that may require operation can occur during pregnancy; fortunately, this happens only rarely. The most common indication for surgery is fulminating colitis-toxic megacolon syndrome, a complication that frequently requires an emergency total colectomy. The outlook for the mother is much better than for the fetus, although some maternal deaths have occurred in years past. Total colectomy with ileostomy in a pregnant patient is technically a very difficult procedure. Fortunately, if the need for operation arises late in the third trimester, modern techniques for the management of prematurity may allow for caeserean section and delivery of a viable infant at an earlier stage than in previous years. Colectomy can be performed at the same time as the delivery or soon after. This has been done on a number of occasions with success both for mother and infant. Surgery for toxic megacolon and other complications of colonic IBD has also been performed on a number of occasions during the earlier stages of pregnancy, but the chances of a live birth from that pregnancy are probably less than 50%. Again, more errors have been made by not operating promptly when the need has arisen than by proceeding prematurely. In fact, the medical emergency presents as much or more of a hazard to the fetus than does the operation.

SMALL INTESTINAL AND ILEOCOLONIC CROHN'S DISEASE

Obstruction, perforation, and sepsis are the most frequent complications of small intestinal or ileocolonic Crohn's disease requiring operation in the pregnant patient, just as in the nonpregnant patient. Although most women whose disease is quiescent at the beginning of pregnancy are likely to remain in remission, sufficient trouble can occur during the course of pregnancy to require operation. Surgery has been performed successfully on many occasions, but at least a 50% incidence of spontaneous abortion and prematurity has followed, about the same level of risk entailed with colectomy for colonic IBD in pregnancy. On the other hand, delay for the sake of the baby poses undue risks to the mother and is usually futile, since the acute abdominal condition for which operation is necessary may threaten the baby just as much or more than the operation.

There have been several cases of pregnant women who were unable to eat because of obstructing Crohn's disease and who were managed successfully during several weeks of later pregnancy with in-hospital or home TPN. In one instance, a patient already on home parenteral nutrition because of otherwise unmanageable complications became pregnant and gave birth to a healthy child.

SUMMARY

Since IBD frequently occurs in young women, it is not surprising that issues related to pregnancy and childbirth arise during the course of disease. The postoperative patient who is cured or in remission is not likely to experience IBD problems related to the pregnancy, and the outlook for the baby is optimistic. Complications that arise and may require operation during pregnancy are serious but usually can be managed successfully.

37 // Surgery in Older People

The risks of operating on the elderly patient are far less than they were a decade ago. In fact, the presence of IBD is not a significant risk factor for the older patient facing surgery of any type. More and more frequently, patients in their 60s and 70s are routinely undergoing major surgical procedures for diseases of all types. "Chronologic age" is now less important than "physiologic age," as measured by a variety of tests of heart, lung, liver, and kidney function. These tests help the physician determine any potential deficiencies in vital functions that may make surgery more risky.

Regardless, at any age, the outcome of surgery is significantly better when it is planned than when it is done as an emergency. Only rarely does IBD have its onset after age 60 or 70 years; most older people with IBD have had their disease for several decades, and are being treated regulary by a physician. Continuing care makes it less likely to develop life-threatening complications.

SURGERY RELATED TO IBD

Some older patients with a long history of ulcerative colitis will no longer have the disease by their late 50s or 60s, having had proctocolectomy and ileostomy some time earlier. They will no longer be on steroids, their nutritional state will be good, and there will be no chronic inflammation to complicate subsequent surgery. Moreover, ileostomy care will be second nature by this time, and they will have no further worry about having surgery for IBD.

Most older people with long-term ulcerative colitis still have their colons—and their disease—and their risk of colon cancer is increased. Periodic colonoscopic examinations with multiple colon biopsies are the best means to detect precancerous changes in the lining of the colon at any age. If these changes are found in elderly patients, experience has shown that total proctocolectomy and ileostomy are *still* the procedures of choice. Alternative operations such as the ileoanal anastomosis or continent ileostomy are not tolerated as well by older people and are not generally performed in this age group. Creation of a standard ileostomy is less likely to be complicated or to require surgical revision, and permits a much more rapid return to daily living and normal activities.

181

Although it is rare, an attack of fulminant ulcerative colitis in an older patient poses a more life-threatening emergency than it does in a younger individual, and prompt surgery is indicated. The key to successful surgery in the elderly person with IBD is not to risk complications that drain his/her limited reserves by delaying major but appropriate surgery.

Just as in the younger patient, Crohn's disease is persistent and recurrent. It usually can be controlled medically and need not interfere with nutrition or the enjoyment of normal activities. A major exacerbation of Crohn's disease is always possible and when it occurs, it is just as likely to respond to vigorous but conservative medical or surgical treatment as in a younger person. The onset of "new" Crohn's colitis in an older individual may represent an exacerbation of long-established but unrecognized Crohn's disease, or, more frequently, it may be a condition known as ischemic colitis masquerading as IBD. In this case, correct diagnosis is essential so that the appropriate therapy can be recommended.

In the elderly person with Crohn's disease, in whom all or part of the colon remains, the risk of colon cancer is greater than that of the general population, but less than that with ulcerative colitis. Nevertheless, the same surveillance measures used in ulcerative colitis should be employed periodically. Cancer of the colon or small intestine in Crohn's disease usually can be controlled by a limited resection, and does not necessarily require proctocolectomy and ileostomy.

SURGERY UNRELATED TO IBD

Does the presence of IBD affect the outcome of unrelated surgery in patients over 60 years? IBD, in itself, does not pose a significant operative risk. Many older IBD patients may have well-controlled ileal or colonic disease with adequate nutritional status. Modern parenteral and enteral techniques allow nutritionally deficient patients of all types to reach a more satisfactory nutritional level before having elective surgery. This recent advance has further increased the safety of elective surgical procedures for the older population. Before any operation, antibacterial agents are used to prevent infection and intravenous steroids may be prescribed to help the patient over the physical stress of surgery. Patients with IBD who are chronically maintained on immunosuppressive drugs such as prednisone might be at a greater risk for infection. However, this risk is not obviously greater than that in other patients treated with steroids, such as those with rheumatoid arthritis, many of whom undergo frequent operations for joint replacement.

Although physiologic age itself can be a risk factor for increased morbidity and mortality in surgery, IBD does not add significantly to that risk. Recent advances in preoperative risk evaluation, patient monitoring, and nutritional and antibiotic support have combined to diminish any effects of age and IBD on the outcome of surgery.

Afterword: Looking to the Future

More than 50 years of experience with IBD justifies a thoughtful and hopeful look into the future. Much has been learned about ulcerative colitis and Crohn's disease in the past half century. We have learned that ulcerative colitis and Crohn's disease are not only disorders of the gastrointestinal tract but that their complications also affect other body systems. We have become increasingly aware of the important role of body defenses and familial tendencies as factors in illness, and have come to appreciate the importance of the gastrointestinal tract in the immune defense against various diseases. Physicians and other health professionals have learned better ways of caring for the IBD patient medically, surgically, and psychologically, and the outlook for the IBD patient has thereby been greatly improved. The importance of controlled clinical studies to evaluate new treatments is well accepted.

POSSIBLE PATHOGENESIS OF IBD

Is it possible now, after a half century of basic and clinical research, to formulate a plausible concept of IBD, a "working hypothesis?" The answer is yes. Ulcerative colitis and Crohn's disease are different yet related diseases. They share many features and sometimes are difficult to tell apart.

The inflammatory process in both ulcerative colitis and Crohn's disease probably begins with a silent or obvious intestinal infection in an individual with a genetic tendency to respond abnormally. Other possibilities include either an unusual reaction to the bacterial population within the bowel, or sensitization of the gut to various bacterial, viral, or dietary antigens early in life. Conceivably, the intestinal and colonic defenses are damaged, perhaps by a genetic defect in the ability of the gut's immune system to limit inflammation. This defect and injury then could result in an increased vulnerability to a variety of subsequent events such as infections or stress.

Thus, it is accepted that inciting events probably cause a diminished capacity of the intestinal mucosal system to defend against a variety of damaging agents, which then initiate the characteristic tissue reactions of IBD (*See Fig. 1, Chapter*

1). Why the tissue reaction in ulcerative colitis and in Crohn's disease persists remains a mystery.

FUTURE RESEARCH POSSIBILITIES

Where then should research efforts be directed in the future? Here are some areas that need further investigation.

Clinical. Cooperative surveys will need to develop and apply standard measures of disease activity and severity to their studies, so that new ideas and new treatment possibilities can be tested in a more uniform fashion throughout the world.

Epidemiology. More extensive national and international cooperative studies must be organized by the CCFA, the International Organization for the Study of Inflammatory Bowel Disease (IOIBD), and selected medical centers throughout the world, to help identify possible environmental factors contributing to IBD.

Microbiology/Virology. Studies are needed to evaluate the possible roles of new bacteria, viruses, and their metabolic products in causing bowel inflammation.

Natural and Experimental Animal Models of IBD. Animal models of ulcerative colitis and Crohn's disease should be developed to test new ideas about the cause of IBD and in evaluating new therapies.

Central Nervous System/Gut Interactions. We need to develop an assay for intestinal neuroendocrine peptides (hormones triggered by the brain and released in the intestine) in an attempt to clarify the psychological relationship between the brain and the gut, and perhaps to help explain the role of stress in IBD.

Nature of IBD Tissue Inflammation. The roles of inflammatory mediators, irritating chemicals released in the gut by cells of the immune system, must be clarified. Knowledge of these mediators and their role in IBD may help to identify new medications to suppress the inflammatory reaction.

Immunology and Gut Defenses. Clarification of the normal immune regulation of small and large bowel is critical to the understanding of the nature of the IBD problem. IBD researchers must study the various immune and physicochemical mechanisms that provide a barrier to injurious agents. This may help to identify new approaches to strengthen the bowel against disease.

Genetic. We need to unravel the mystery of the genetic susceptibility to IBD and how genes govern the immune defenses and response of the GI tract.

Therapy. We must develop more effective nutritional supports, stronger and safer antibiotics to control gut bacteria, and more effect antiinflammatory agents to inhibit the formation of damaging chemical substances. Also on the horizon are drugs to improve the integrity of the bowel wall, antiviral compounds, more agents that modulate the immune response, and measures for strengthening host defenses. The hopeful aspect of these suggestions is that each is possible.

Finally, is it realistic, after these many years, to expect the cause or causes of ulcerative colitis and Crohn's disease to be discovered in the near future? Again, the answer is yes. Particularly impressive is the rising public interest in IBD, the gradually increasing support of research, the important supportive role of the CCFA, and the growing numbers of better trained clinicians and investigators interested in IBD; all greatly increase the possibility of successful research.

Inflammatory bowel diseases are one of the major clinical problems in medicine today. Clarification of their cause will increase our understanding not only of gastrointestinal function in health and disease, but also of other medical problems beyond the gastrointestinal tract.

Joseph B. Kirsner, M.D., Ph.D.
Chairman Emeritus
National Scientific Advisory Committee
Crohn's & Colitis Foundation of America, Inc.

Glossary of Medical Terms

abscess: a pocket or collection of pus. In IBD these typically form in the abdominal cavity or rectal area.

ankylosis: fusion of the bones of the spinal column.

anticholinergic: a class of drugs that relax the smooth muscle of the intestine.

autoimmunity: an inflammatory reaction to one's own tissues.

clinical: involving the direct observation and treatment of patients.

contraindication: any circumstance making a form of medical or surgical treatment unadvisable.

dermatitis: irritation or inflammation of the skin.

edema: accumulation of excessive amounts of fluid in the tissues that may result in swelling.

electrolytes: acids, bases, and salts essential for maintaining life.

endoscopy: direct examination of the interior of the digestive tract using a fiberoptic endoscope, such as a sigmoidoscope, colonoscope, or gastroscope.

epidemiology: the study of the frequency and distribution of diseases in the population.

exacerbation: an increase in symptoms or reactivation of disease; a relapse.

fissure: a crack or crevice in the skin surrounding the anus.

fistula: an abnormal channel connecting two structures, e.g., adjacent loops of intestine or the intestine and another structure such as the bladder, vagina, or skin.

fluoroscopy: a type of x-ray examination in which the shadows of organs being examined are made visible on a screen.

folic acid: one of the vitamins responsible for the formation of red blood cells. Folic acid deficiency may occur in IBD patients, especially in those taking sulfasalazine.

fulminant: with extreme rapidity.

gut: general word for intestine or bowel.

idiopathic: of unknown cause.

immunology: study of the body's immune response to disease.

immunosuppressive agents: drugs that suppress the body's immune response to disease or environmental agents.

inflammation: a process characterized by pain, redness, heat, and swelling.

inflammatory mediators: powerful chemicals released by the body as part of the inflammatory response.

intractable: unrelieved by medical treatment.

lactose intolerance: a condition caused by a decrease or absence of the enzyme lactase, which aids in digestion of milk sugar.

leukotrienes: powerful chemical mediators released during the inflammatory process that promote the migration of white blood cells to the site of inflammation.

lumen: the interior of a hollow organ, such as the intestine.

mucus: a whitish substance normally produced by the intestine and that may be found in increased amounts in the stool when the intestine is diseased.

osteonecrosis: death of bone tissue. This may result from use of long-term high-dose steroids.

oxalate stones: kidney stones formed from calcium oxalate, and found in IBD patients with fat malabsorption resulting from ileal disease or resection.

oxygen radicals: toxic products of oxygen metabolism that may cause tissue damage in IBD.

paresthesias: abnormal sensations in the feet and lower legs, often felt as "pins and needles."

pathogen: a microorganism (bacterium or virus) capable of causing disease.

pathogenesis: the origin and development of disease.

perineal: involving the anal and genital areas and their surrounding tissues.

prolapse: the falling or protrusion of an organ, such as the rectum or stoma.

prostaglandin: another inflammatory mediator that may cause the intestine to lose fluid and electrolytes.

protein losing enteropathy: loss of circulating proteins and other nutrients through the inflamed bowel wall.

remission: a reduction of symptoms and a return to good health.

sepsis: infection of the bloodstream with microorganisms.

spondylitis: arthritis of the spine.

thrombophlebitis: inflammation and clotting of veins.

Glossary of Surgical Terms

adhesions: scar tissue. In IBD these often connect two adjacent loops of intestine or a section of intestine to the abdominal wall.

anastomosis: a surgical connection.

catheter: a thin tube placed into a body cavity, organ, or vessel for the purpose of administering or draining fluids.

colectomy: removal of part or all of the colon.

colostomy: a surgically created opening of the colon to the abdominal wall, allowing the diversion of fecal waste.

distal: closer to the anus; downstream.

drains: catheters placed around areas where bowel has been removed to collect and drain fluids and prevent wound infection.

excision: surgical removal.

hemorrhage: abnormally heavy bleeding.

ileostomy: a surgically created opening of the ileum to the abdominal wall, allowing the diversion of fecal waste.

ileus: temporary paralysis of bowel, often resulting from surgery, abdominal infection, or electrolyte imbalance.

nasogastric tube: a thin, flexible tube passed through the nose or mouth into the stomach. This tube is necessary to aspirate fluids and air that collect in the stomach when the bowel is obstructed or after intestinal surgery.

obstruction: a blockage of the small or large intestine preventing the normal passage of intestinal contents.

percutaneous: through the skin.

perforation: formation of a hole in the bowel wall, allowing intestinal contents to enter the peritoneal cavity.

peristalsis: wave-like muscular movements that propel food through the digestive tract.

peristomal: the area immediately surrounding the stoma.

peritoneum: the membrane that encloses the abdominal organs, forming the peritoneal or abdominal cavity.

peritonitis: inflammation of the peritoneum, usually resulting from an intestinal perforation.

proctectomy: removal of the rectum.

proctocolectomy: removal of the entire colon and rectum.

proximal: closer to the mouth; upstream.

resection: surgical removal of a diseased portion of intestine.

reservoir: a surgically created pouch made from the distal ileum to collect intestinal waste.

sphincter: a ring of muscle tissue keeping certain sections of the digestive tract (such as the anus) closed.

stenosis: a narrowing.

stoma: a surgically created opening of the bowel onto the skin, the result of ostomy surgery.

stricture: a narrowed area of intestine caused by active inflammation or scar tissue.

subtotal colectomy: removal of part or most of the colon, leaving a part (usually the rectum) intact.

sutures: materials used in surgery to rejoin cut tissues and close wounds.

Bibliography

Alexander-Williams J, Allan A, Morel P, Hawker P C, Dykes P W, O'Connor H. The therapeutic dilation of enteric strictures due to Crohn's disease. *Ann Royal Coll Surg* 1986;68:95–97.

Biddle W L, Greenberger N J, Swan J T, McPhee M S, Miner P B Jr. 5-aminosalicylic acid enemas: Effective agent in maintaining remission in left-sided ulcerative colitis. *Gastroenterology* 1988;94(4):1075–1079.

Brandt L J. Colitis in the elderly. *Hosp Prac* 1987;22:165–191.

Brandt L J, Bernstein L H, Boley S J. Metronidazole therapy for perineal Crohn's disease: A follow-up study. *Gastroenterology* 1982;83:383–387.

Cohen Z. Current status of the continent ileostomy. *Canad J Surg* 1987;30(5):357–358.

Daum F. Pediatric inflammatory bowel disease. In: Silverberg M, Daum F (eds). *Textbook of Pediatric Gastroenterology, 2nd Ed.* Chicago: Year Book Medical Publishers, 1988:392–418.

Drossman D A. Psychosocial aspects of ulcerative colitis and Crohn's disease. In: Kirsner J B, Shorter R G (eds). *Inflammatory Bowel Disease*. Philadelphia: Lea & Febiger, 1988:209–226.

Fazio V W, Galandink S. Strictureplasty in diffuse Crohn's jejunoileitis. *Dis Colon Rectum* 1985;28(7):512–518.

Friedman G. Treatment of refractory proctosigmoiditis and left-sided colitis with a rectally instilled non-glucocorticoid, non-mineralocorticoid steroid. *Gastroenterology* 1985;88(5):1388.

Glotzer D J. The surgical management of idiopathic inflammatory bowel disease. In: Kirsner J B, Shorter R G (eds). *Inflammatory Bowel Disease*. Philadelphia: Lea & Febiger, 1988:585–644.

Goldstein F. Immunosuppressant therapy of inflammatory bowel disease: Pharmacologic and clinical aspects (Review article). *J Clin Gastroenterol* 1987;9(6):654–658.

Greenstein A J, Janowitz H D, Sachar D B. The extra-intestinal complications of Crohn's disease and ulcerative colitis: A study of 700 patients. *Medicine* 1976;55(4):401–412.

Greenstein A J, Mann D, Sachar D B, Aufses A H. Free perforation in Crohn's disease: A survey of 99 cases. *Am J Gastroenterol* 1985;80:682–689.

Janowitz H D. The "natural history" of inflammatory bowel disease and therapeutic decisions (1986 Stuart Distinguished Lecture). *Am J Gastroenterol* 1987;82(6):498–503.

MacDermott R P, Stenson W F. The immunology of idiopathic inflammatory bowel disease. *Hosp Prac* 1986;97–116.

Meyers S, Sachar D B, Goldberg J D, Janowitz H D. Corticotropin vs hydrocortisone in the intravenous treatment of ulcerative colitis: A prospective, randomized double-blind clinical trial. *Gastroenterology* 1983;85(2):351–357.

Korelitz B I. Pregnancy, fertility, and inflammatory bowel disease. *Am J Gastroenterol* 1985;80:365–370.

Motil K J, Grand R J. Nutritional management of inflammatory bowel disease (Review article). *Ped Clin N Am* 1985;32(2):447–469.

Oakley J R, Jagelman D G, Fazio V W, Lavery I C, Weakley F L, Easley K, Farmer R G. Complications and quality of life after ileorectal anastomosis for ulcerative colitis. *Am J Surg* 1985;149(1):23–30.

Pemberton J H, Kelly K A, Beart R W Jr, Dozois R R, Wolff B G, Ilstrup D M. Ileal pouch-anal anastomosis for chronic ulcerative colitis: Long-term results. *Ann Surg* 1987;206(4):504–513.

Peppercorn M A. Sulfasalazine: Pharmacology, clinical use, toxicity and related new drug development. *Ann Intern Med* 1984;3:337.

Present D H, Kelly K A. Executive Summary of NFIC's Ileostomy Alternatives Workshop. *IBD News* 1987;8(1):1–3.

Rosenberg I H, Bengoa J M, Sitrin M D. Nutritional aspects of inflammatory bowel disease. *Ann Rev Nutr* 1985;5:463–484.

Sachar D B. Placebo-controlled trials in gastroenterology: A position paper of The American College of Gastroenterology. *Am J Gastroenterol* 1984;79(12):913–917.

Sachar D B, Wolfson D M, Greenstein A J, Goldberg J, Janowitz H D. Risk factors for postoperative recurrence in Crohn's disease. *Gastroenterology* 1983;85:917–921.

Sales D J, Kirsner J B. The prognosis of inflammatory bowel disease. *Arch Intern Med* 1983;143(2): 294–299.

Schorr-Lesnick B, Brandt L J. Selected rheumatologic and dermatologic manifestations of inflammatory bowel disease. *Am J Gastroenterol* 1988;83(3):216–223.

Schroeder K W, Tremaine W J, Ilstrup D M. Coated oral 5-aminosalicylic acid therapy for mildly to moderately active ulcerative colitis: A randomized study. *N Eng J Med* 1987;317(26):1625–1629.

Sohn N, Korelitz B I. Local operative treatment of anorectal Crohn's disease. *J Clin Gastroenterol* 1982;4:395–399.

Strauss R E. Ocular manifestations of Crohn's disease: Literature review. *Mt Sinai J Med* 1988;55: 353–356.

Subject Index

Index compiled by June G. Rosenberg, Reference Librarian, Nathan Cummings Center Medical Library, Memorial Sloan–Kettering Cancer Center, New York.